THE MENTAL HEALTH
CONSULTATION FIELD

TM

THE MENTAL HEALTH
CONSULTATION FIELD

Edited by

Saul Cooper, M.A.

Washtenaw County Community Mental Health Center
Ann Arbor, Michigan

William F. Hodges, Ph.D.

University of Colorado
Boulder, Colorado

Volume XI, *Community Psychology Series*
American Psychological Association,
Division 27
Series Editor: Bernard L. Bloom, Ph.D.

Sponsored by Division of Community Psychology

American Psychological Association

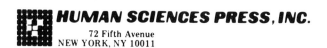 **HUMAN SCIENCES PRESS, INC.**
72 Fifth Avenue
NEW YORK, NY 10011

Printed in the United States of America
23456789 987654321

Library of Congress Cataloging in Publication Data
Main entry under title:

The Mental health consultation field.

    (Community psychology series, ISSN 0731-0471 ; 11)
    Includes index.
1. Psychiatric consultation. 2. Community mental
health services. I. Cooper, Saul, 1927-
II. Hodges, William F. III. Series.
RC455.2.C65M45   1983   362.2'04256   83-197
ISBN 0-89885-130-0

TITLES IN THE COMMUNITY PSYCHOLOGY SERIES
UNDER THE EDITORSHIP OF DANIEL ADELSON,
FOUNDING SERIES EDITOR
(1972-1979)

Volume 1: Man as the Measure: The Crossroads, edited by Daniel Adelson

Volume 2: The University and the Urban Crisis, edited by Howard E.Mitchell

Volume 3: Psychological Stress in the Campus Community: Theory, Research and Action, edited by Bernard L. Bloom

Volume 4: Psychology of the Planned Community: The New Town Experience, edited by Donald C. Klein

Volume 5: Challenges to the Criminal Justice System: The Perspectives of Community Psychology, edited by Theodore R. Sarbin

UNDER THE EDITORSHIP OF BERNARD L. BLOOM

Volume 6: Paraprofessionals in the Human Services, edited by Stanley S. Robin and Morton O. Wagenfeld

Volume 7: Psychiatric Patient Rights and Patient Advocacy: Issues and Evidence, edited by Bernard L. Bloom and Shirley J. Asher

Volume 8: Assessing Health and Human Service Needs: Concepts, Methods, and Applications, edited by Roger A. Bell, Martin Sundel, Joseph F. Aponte, Stanley A. Murrell, and Elizabeth Lin

Volume 9: The Pluralistic Society, edited by Stanley Sue and Thom Moore

Volume 10: The Self-Help Revolution, edited by Alan Gartner and Frank Riessman

Volume 11: The Mental Health Consultation Field, edited by Saul Cooper and William F. Hodges

THE COMMUNITY PSYCHOLOGY SERIES
SPONSORED BY
THE DIVISION OF COMMUNITY PSYCHOLOGY
OF THE
AMERICAN PSYCHOLOGICAL ASSOCIATION

The Community Psychology Series has as its central purpose the building of philosophic, theoretical, scientific, and empirical foundations for action research in the community and in its subsystems and for education and training for such action research.

As a publication of the Division of Community Psychology, the series is particularly concerned with the development of community psychology as a subarea of psychology. It emphasizes in general application and integration of theories and findings from other areas of psychology and in particular development of community psychology methods, theories, and principles as these stem from actual community research and practice.

CONTENTS

CONTRIBUTORS

SAUL COOPER is director of the Washtenaw County Community Mental Health Center in Ann Arbor, Michigan. He is adjunct professor of psychology at the University of Michigan.

LEONARD D. GOODSTEIN is president of University Associates, a San Diego-based publishing and consulting firm. He is author of *Consulting with Human Service Systems.*

BENJAMIN H. GOTTLIEB is associate professor of psychology, University of Guelph, Ontario.

KENNETH HELLER is professor of psychology at the University of Indiana and is coauthor of *Psychology and Community Change.*

WILLIAM F. HODGES is associate professor of psychology at the University of Colorado, Boulder, where he is director of clinical training.

JAMES G. KELLY is professor of psychology at the University of Illinois, Chicago Circle.

DONALD C. KLEIN was project director of the Pilot Conference on Primary Prevention. He is currently professor and coordinator of an applied behavioral sciences graduate program at Johns Hopkins University. He is author of *Community Dynamics and Mental Health.*

TIMOTHY G. KUEHNEL AND JULIE M. KUEHNEL are assistant research psychologists in the Department of Psychiatry and Biobehavioral Sciences, Camarillo/Neuropsychiatric Institute Research Program, University of California at Los Angeles—School of Medicine.

RONALD LIPPITT is president of Human Resource Development and Associates and is recently coauthor of *The Consulting Process in Action.*

PHILIP A. MANN is a school psychologist with Area Education Agency 7, Cedar Falls, Iowa. He is author of *Community Psychology: Concepts and Applications.*

13

FORTUNE V. MANNINO is at the Mental Health Study Center, National Institute of Mental Health. He is coeditor of *The Practice of Mental Health Consultation.*

NOEL A. MAZADE is program director with the Staff College, National Institute of Mental Health, in Rockville, Maryland, specializing in management training for and consultation to senior mental health program managers.

JOHN MONAHAN is professor of law at the University of Virginia, Charlottesville. He is coauthor of *Psychology and Community Change.*

RICHARD A. SCHMUCK is professor of educational psychology at the University of Oregon. He is coauthor of *The Second Handbook of Organizational Development in Schools* and the third edition of *Group Processes in Education.*

MILTON F. SHORE is at the Mental Health Study Center, National Institute of Mental Health. He is coeditor of *The Practice of Mental Health Consultation* and currently president of the American Orthopsychiatric Association.

PREFACE

Although the term *consultation* has a long history, the use of that word in the phrase *mental health consultation* is a relatively recent one, dating to the years immediately prior to establishment of the community mental health movement in the early 1960s.

Mental health consultation is an indirect service; that is, it constitutes an interaction in which one person—the consultant—is asked to be of help to other persons—consultees—in regard to a work problem pertinent to a human services client. In development of the intellectual foundation of the community mental health movement, mental health consultation was perhaps the single most innovative technology that was introduced into the practitioner's list of skills.

The hopes for mental health consultation included its multiplicative or spread effect upon the field, in that consultants could influence consultees, who, in turn, could influence clients; its role in primary prevention, in that clients in other systems, such as students in public schools, might become less vulnerable to life stresses because of the consultation received by teachers; its potential positive influence upon many phases of the professional lives of consultees; and its role in making consultants wiser, by familiarizing them with the life and work of a wide variety of consultees and clients with whom consultants might not ordinarily interact.

Yet there has always been a curious ambivalence about mental health consultation as a rigorous set of skills. Although almost no mental health practitioners undertake direct service to clients without prior training, relatively few mental health consultants have been trained in mental health consultation. Although most psychotherapists have some form of ongoing supervision of their clinical work, it is the rare agency that provides supervision for mental health consultation. Although entire volumes are based upon carefully dissected interactions between a client and a psychotherapist, almost no such written materials are published for training in mental health consultation. Indeed, far too little is written about mental health consultation.

This volume, edited by two superbly qualified community psychologists, is a significant addition to the mental health consultation literature. It represents an effort to strengthen the conceptual base of mental health con-

15

sultation by examining its functional models, by identifying and considering many of the issues of central concern to mental health consultants, and by considering the future of mental health consultation. I am delighted to have this work part of the Community Psychology Series.

Bernard L. Bloom
Boulder, Colorado

Part I

INTRODUCTION

Chapter 1

GENERAL INTRODUCTION

William F. Hodges, Ph.D.
Saul Cooper, M.A.

The community mental health consultation field has evolved into an exciting strategy for indirect service to individuals in the community and for community change. From its initial conceptualizations in the 1960s to the present, mental health consultation has developed from bootstrap learning-by-doing to a federally mandated service of comprehensive mental health centers—an extraordinary change in such a short time. This brief history has not been without trauma and discouragement. Orientation toward one-to-one psychotherapy as a way of handling a community's mental health problems has so embued our society that mental health professionals and community leaders have been reluctant to develop consultation services when the "real" (familiar) intervention is available. Funding has been difficult when community members receive service only indirectly. Conceptualization of guiding principles has been slow in evolving. Gerald Caplan's book (1970) formed the early organization of consultation into the familiar processes of client-centered case consultation, consultee-centered case consultation, program-centered administrative consultation, and consultee-centered administrative consultation. Although some recent writings have gone beyond this conceptualization, most are summaries of Caplan's models. Conceptual development since that time has grown by bits and pieces. It is the purpose of this text to bring together leading thinkers in the mental health consultation field to summarize ways in which consultation can be conceptualized.

Community mental health consultation can be defined as the process by which a mental health professional interacts with community-based professionals and other service providers (the consultees) to supply information, skill training, and individual-process change or system change in order to help the consultee or the system better serve the mental health needs of the people in the community. There is no client in the traditional sense. The consultant provides potential help, but not direct service, to the people in the community. The consultant works with those people who serve the community directly, the teachers, police, nurses, welfare workers, recreational aides, etc., by helping them more effectively work with individuals in the community in terms of their mental health or work with the community system itself, which is made up of those individuals. It is customary in books such as this one to differentiate community mental health consultation from supervision, teaching, and therapy. Readers unfamiliar with such distinctions should refer to earlier summaries of the field (Altrocchi, 1972). Suffice it to say that such distinctions are critical, and the beginning consultant should have those differences and their implications clearly in mind.

The basic purpose of this book is to provide the conceptualization of the process of consultation so that the practitioner and student can (1) understand the dimensions that structure the role, (2) monitor what he or she is doing, and (3) decide how to improve in order to be more effective.

We should make very clear that consultation is not education in the traditional sense, even though consultation and education are often lumped together in the same unit of a mental health center. Education per se differs from consultation in that education is essentially provision of information that one thinks might be useful to someone in a particular position. Consultation, in contrast, is tailored to the needs of the individual consultee, and those needs by definition must evolve into one's assessment of the consultee's knowledge, skill, as well as individual process or system process. Thus, consultation, like education, involves change, but differs from education in three basic ways: (1) the degree to which it is individualized to a person and a system, (2) degree to which the focus will change as a function of the interaction with the person and the system, and (3) the basic underlying philosophy.

PHILOSOPHICAL ORIENTATION OF CONSULTATION

The community mental health center movement has as its base the assumption of response to community needs. Community mental health consultation is embedded in the community mental health movement both as a strategy of intervention and as a philosophy of helping communities.

The basic focus of consultation is to share competence and power, to increase the competence of the community to solve its own problems and improve the quality of living. Since the focus is to decrease dependency by increasing competence, the constant orientation of the community mental health consultant is always to move toward reducing the need for the consultant, to "talk oneself out of a job." Implicit in community mental health consultation is a philosophical orientation toward healthy systems and healthy communities, an orientation toward primary prevention by either removing the stressors in the community or immunizing the people in the community against those stressors (Bloom, 1971, 1979).

It is seductive for the consultant to take over the problem of the consultee, both to increase one's own self-worth, by demonstrating that one knows more than the consultee, and to be efficient. Such an approach increases dependency and does not encourage people within the system to change. Since the basic orientation is to give away competence, the consultant uses every opportunity to share that power and competence. When a teacher wants a consultant to have a conference with a difficult parent, the effective consultant is likely to refuse. The consultant might agree to see the parent with the teacher, to discuss strategy before the meeting, and to meet afterward to determine if the teacher and the consultant accomplished what they set out to do. In this way the consultant can teach the consultee to handle upset parents, to reduce the adversarial nature of teacher-parent conferences, and to explore techniques for increasing collaboration between teacher and parent concerning plans for helping the child. To take over the role of conferee with parents would change nothing in the consultee or system permanently. Although helping another person is seldom inappropriate and has value in and of itself, the mental health consultant has the higher-order goal of changing the system to be more responsive to the needs of the people it serves.

The first part of this book is on models of consultation. What are the guiding orientations toward helping people that determine what the consultant does? What are the implications of a particular orientation, and how do the various orientations interact?

The second part is focused on particular issues that affect the day-to-day life of the consultant. Entry, transfer, and termination are transition times in consultation. Accountability is becoming an increasing concern. Also discussed are strategies for generating funds, a difficult problem given the direct nature of the service. Ethics are a serious problem when one is providing a service to one person in order to help someone else. Even more serious ethical implications are involved in community psychology when not everyone in a community may participate or approve of a change. Finally, consultation as an issue of political power is discussed.

In the third part, the authors look to the future of consultation. If consultation is embedded in a philosophy of change, then consultation itself must evolve into other processes for helping people. Self-help networks and human service networks are two such evolutionary products that are being seen today. Finally, limitations to effectiveness in consultation today and speculations about future opportunities are discussed.

TRAINING AS A CONSULTANT

This is not a how-to-do-it book. It is our belief that such a book would not be very effective. Consultation requires knowledge and skill. One does not, however, learn skill by simply reading about a process, any more than a person learns to do psychotherapy by listening to a lecture.

The consultant must, of course, have information about mental health concepts and an understanding of principles of behavior of individuals and systems. Effective intervention based on that knowledge is a significant skill, however. Many mental health professionals are very knowledgeable about mental health concepts, but ineffective in translating these concepts into useful intervention in the community. Attempts to train consultants by means of didactic courses have been generally ineffective. Professionals do not increase involvement in a role simply because they have heard about it. It has been our extensive experience that the most effective way of increasing the skill of consultation is through modeling, by working with someone working in the role of consultant. The bootstrap technique for learning consultation can work, but it is risky and does not build on the experience of others who have worked out the conceptualizations that guide behavior. The early ideas on consultation were hard-learned and filled with mistakes. Doing it on your own has the danger of, at best, "*re*inventing the wheel" and, at worse, "*not* inventing the wheel."

CONTINUED SUPERVISION

Many occupations in which consultees find themselves are lonely. The jobs of the elementary school teacher, the single patrol officer on the police force, and the community public health nurse are all lonely jobs. One important service that the community mental health consultant can provide to such individuals is significant emotional support.

Most consultants, whether working in a consultation and education (C and E) unit of a community mental health center or in private practice, are also in a lonely profession. C and E units are typically understaffed and underfunded (for reasons why, see the chapter on accountability and funding by Shore and Mannino). All privately practicing professionals are typically isolated in their work, but particularly so are consultants because of the stressful nature of consultation.

We want to remind the reader that consultation is significantly different from psychotherapy in day-to-day practice. The therapist waits in the office until the client arrives; the process begins again, without basic change, with the next client. With repeated contacts with the same client, the life of the therapist becomes reasonably predictable. One frequently knows ahead of time which clients are going to be enjoyable or difficult and in what ways. As we have indicated, in the day-to-day life of the mental health consultant, change characterizes the day: change in the system and in the person-environment interaction. This change makes consultation exciting but also significantly stressful.

We have found that one lowers the stress, reduces the isolation, and the quality of the activity enhanced by combining consultation with training. We prefer to take a consultation student along. When the consultant explains his/her understanding of a problem and the reasons why a particular strategy was used, the consultant may discover conceptualizations of the system that might not have occurred otherwise. Feedback based on observations has a high learning value.

We have also found that peer supervision groups are highly effective means of maintaining and raising skills. Even one hour a week of peer group supervision is effective in forcing the consultants to think about what they are doing, to conceptualize the individual consultee and the system, to share competences, and to enhance their own roles.

RESEARCH

As you read the chapters in this book, you may be struck by the lack of research supporting the views of the various authors. Most of the references are conceptualizations of practitioners. Unfortunately research has seldom been done to answer questions of cost-effectiveness or cost-benefit ratios. Mannino and Shore also wrote a review of the literature on change in consultation (1975) and concluded that in 70 percent of the cases some evidence of change in the consultee, client, or system was evident. Inspection of the studies gives a less optimistic view of the evidence supporting the effectiveness of consultation. Results vary from one study to the next, and the level of change, whether at the individual consultee, client, or system level, is difficult to predict.

All the problems generated by psychotherapy research, questions of operationalization of concepts, variability of treatment, and disagreement on treatment goals are compounded in consultation research. Change in the consultee could be measured in self-concept, knowledge, job-related skills, job satisfaction, or attitudes toward mental health or toward the client or job. Changes in the client could focus on maladjustment, misbehavior (or target behavior), self-concept, or perceived quality of life. Changes in the system are almost unlimited in scope: support, communication, power, competence, openness, tolerance, or quality of life. Since by our definition consultation shifts levels, from education to consultee process and then to system process over time, evaluation becomes extremely difficult.

EVALUATION AS AN INTERVENTION STRATEGY

Let us encourage consultants to use program evaluation as an accompanying tool of intervention. One of the editors routinely asked elementary school teachers to rate the behavior of cases at the time of referral and at the end of the school year. One year he also obtained beginning- and end-of-year ratings from nonserved schools concerning children with behavior and emotional problems. Not only did this procedure provide information about which child required continued follow-up, but it also gave information about which types of problems were not helped. In addition, it was possible to relate demographic characteristics to effectiveness. The finding that the program was not helpful (as compared with the nontreated control) for some problems led to new intervention techniques. The finding that, the younger the child, the better consultation effectiveness, gave us justification to move to a prevention model and focus the consultation program in kindergarten and first-grade classes.

TIME

A final comment: In earlier, more affluent times, there was a tendency to change jobs in order to obtain promotions or raises. More recently, economic conditions have led to reduced geographic mobility of mental health professionals, a change that is to the advantage of the community. It has been our experience that the consultant *must* make a significant commitment in terms of time and energy in order to be effective. It may take as long as several years to make an effective entry into a system. This commitment is required in order to obtain the conceptualizations necessary in order to move effectively at different levels of consultation *and* to build the trust in the community required in order to effect change.

Consultation has been reasonably well established as a community care-giving intervention technique. We hope this book enhances the work of students and practitioners so that they may make further contributions to the mental health consultation field.

REFERENCES

Altrocchi, J. Mental health consultation. In S.E. Golann & C. Eisdorfer (Eds.), *Handbook of community mental health.* New York: Appleton-Century-Crofts, 1972.

Bloom, B. L. Strategies for the prevention of mental disorders. In G. Rosenblum (Ed.), *Issues in community psychology and preventive mental health.* New York: Behavioral Publications, 1971.

_____. Prevention of mental disorders: Recent advances in theory and practice. *Community Mental Health Journal,* 1979, *15*(3) 179-191.

Caplan, G. The theory and practice of mental health consultation. New York: Basic Books, 1970.

Mannino, F. V., & Shore, M. F. The effects of consultation. *American Journal of Community Psychology,* March 1975, *3,* 1-21.

Part II

MODELS

Chapter 2

MODELS OF CONSULTATION

William F. Hodges, Ph.D.
Saul Cooper, M.A.

In our review of the consultation literature, we concluded that three basic models of consultation were essential for an understanding of the levels of intervention and basic strategies of intervention: educational, individual-process, and system-process models. Note that these are *models*, not theories, of consultation. *Theories* in mental health are the basic assumptions about the nature of people that lead to particular interventions, such as dynamic, humanistic, or behavioral. Any particular theory of personality may be included under each model, although some correlations between models and theories do occur. We assume that the mental health professional who decides to do community mental health consultation has been well grounded in diagnosis, personality theory, and intervention strategies.

Unlike the theory of personality, the model of consultation is not simply a case of preference. One needs to take a specific stand concerning the levels of intervention and understand why, in this particular case, that level was chosen. Everyone has a model of change, implicit or explicit. If the model (like the theory of personality) is implicit, there is a danger that the person will work inconsistently and may at times work at cross-purpose with himself or herself.

A variety of other authors have included a different number of models. Gerald Caplan (1970) in his pioneering work on consultation included four: client-centered case consultation, consultee-centered case consultation, client-centered administrative consultation, and consultee-centered administrative consultation. These four levels of consultation are not identical to the three we are proposing, but there is some overlap, as will be indicated later. Blake and Mouton (1976) proposed a grid of five units of change, five levels of interventions, and four levels of issues and then organized their

29

book by that systematic approach. Although the present model is not as complex as theirs, it is our belief that the levels of intervention and units of change in their approach can be incorporated into the three models of consultation discussed here.

EDUCATIONAL MODEL

In the educational model, the consultant conceptualizes the difficulty on the part of the consultee in solving a mental health-related problem as due primarily to lack of skill or knowledge. Intervention is focused around modeling skills or imparting information. Typically the consultant using this approach has a behavior modification orientation, but may draw on rational-emotive therapy, Rogerian therapy, dynamic interpretations, or other theoretical orientations.

This model of consultation is similar to what Caplan called *client-centered case consultation,* although he included lack of knowledge or skills under *consultee-centered case consultation.* The educational model has not been the model about which consultation has predominantly been written. Perhaps this lack of interest has been due in part to Caplan's attitude toward the educational model. He clearly had little interest in providing information about how to handle the mental health implications that a client presented to a consultee. He spent few (16) pages of his book on consultation (Caplan, 1970) on client-centered case consultation and many (98) pages on what he saw as the dynamically more interesting consultee-centered case consultation. Yet it is education and information that many consultees are seeking: "How can I handle this problem more effectively?" It would be a mistake, however, to assume that providing a diagnosis and a three- or four-point recommendation is going to be effective in helping the consultee in working better with the client.

Unfortunately, when they provide information to a consultee, consultants tend to forget what they have learned about how people receive information and learn skills. Most mental health professionals have learned that lecture formats are not very useful in teaching strategies of intervention. We would never assume that one could learn psychotherapy by reading a book and yet forget that behaviors such as providing warmth to a client, being sensitive to feelings, rewarding appropriate behavior, ignoring demands for attention, or interpreting a conflict are skills that are learned. Old patterns are habits and are difficult to break. New learning follows well-known principles of behavior modification, reinforcement, and modeling. It is not surprising that the major writings on an educational model of consultation are in the area of behavior modification. The chapter by Timothy and Julie Kuehnel is strongly oriented this way. Their chapter makes clear why non-behavior modifiers have perhaps been less successful with this model of intervention. The naive consultant is all too quick to take learning principles for granted and simply provide information that is not usable in that form. The care with which the Kuehnels develop the *structure* for learning makes it clear that significant thinking must go into how to help the consultee to understand and effectively use a skill.

Just because the educational model of consultation has attracted more behavior modifiers than other theorists does not mean that consultants with other orientations cannot use this model effectively. We have found it useful to translate the theory of Hiam Ginott/Carl Rogers into an effective intervention for grade school teachers. Many children who are significantly withdrawn or shy seem to be anxious because of low self-esteem. These children may not see the world as supportive and accepting. An effective intervention using a Rogerian approach was presented in an educational formulation. When a case was presented that seemed to fit this conceptualization, the teacher was given the following information:

1. Withdrawn children may feel rejected and/or may be repressing significant feelings. If we can help them to express their feelings appropriately, we may be able to help them be more open and spontaneous.

2. Tell the child how he or she feels several times during the day. You can carry out this process while passing the child's desk or in the hall or on the way to the lunchroom. Try to include, at different times, reflection of both positive and negative feelings, if both are present. Use short and non-judgmental phrases. (The consultant should not assume that the teacher understands how people can make reflection of feelings judgmental.)

3. Simply say to the child, "You look bored" or "you seemed to have a lot of fun on the playground today" or "It looks like that assignment really made you angry."

4. Do not use judgmental phrases, such as "...and if you felt that way more often we would all get along better" or "...and if you weren't so angry you would enjoy school more," which are not accepting of feelings.

5. Try not to pause. Children are so used to judgmental statements from teachers that if you allow an expectant pause, the children will fill in the judgmental phrase themselves.

First, note that this approach is basically an educational model. The assumption is that the teacher may be able to use a technique that would be effective in helping an inhibited child to be more expressive. Experience has indicated that a large number of consultees are able to use this advice well when the steps are carefully spelled out (since there is no assumption that the consultee knows how to use this simple intervention). Finally, it should be noted that this intervention has a predictable path that helps the consultee track whether it is helping. At first, the child may respond with surprise or no apparent indication that the behavior on the part of the teacher was meaningful. After about a week or two, the child may spontaneously elaborate on the feeling even though the teacher has not indicated a demand for a response and may be moving on to another child. After several weeks of spontaneous elaboration of day-to-day feelings, the child is more likely to respond with feelings that affect him or her on a deeper level. We had a fifth-grade boy who had not spoken more than single words for the first 4 months in a new school. By getting the teacher to use this technique and working with her to consult with the father (in a single-parent home), within 1 month the boy was chatting freely about his life. This example also suggests that at times providing didactic information, without modeling or role playing, may work better than is implied in the Kuehnels' chapter.

It is presumptuous for a mental health consultant to assume that all consultee failures in helping a client are due to unresolved theme interference or underlying personality dynamics. The mental health consultant is typically rather uninformed about the training and educational background of the consultee with whom he or she is working. Few training programs in non-mental-health professions spend a significant amount of time (or, for that matter, any time at all) applying mental health principles to the population they serve.

An example of how a situation was handled using an educational model, when an individual-dynamics model could have been proposed, follows:

One of the editors was presented with the problem of excessive fighting in the playground at an elementary school. As the consultant collected data on antecedent conditions and consequences, he discovered that the principal was paddling up to 15 boys a day in his office as punishment for the misbehavior. The consultant learned that the principal had been a Golden Gloves champion. It would have been easy to assume that the consultant was presented with a theme-interference problem, however, assuming lack of knowledge, until there was evidence to contradict that assumption, he informed the principal that research indicates that physical punishment seems to increase physical aggression in children, even though many other aspects of punishment are desirable (being close to the misbehavior and short, leaving no residual guilt). The principal was distressed to learn this information (for more than one reason, perhaps) but agreed to try social isolation as a punishment. Fights went from 10 to 15 per play period to 2 to 3 per play period within 1 month. Why was there still a problem? It became apparent that in this small and conservative community, physical punishment as well as encouragement of aggressive behavior ("Don't let anybody push you around.") were common among parents. Such information could lead to a more systemwide approach, which will be discussed later.

It is also presumptuous to assume that the consultee operates on the same system of rewards and intrinsic interests that the consultant has. One consultant was working with a teacher who was trying to get a parent to be more consistent with rewards and punishments. The consultant had the teacher call the parent every day initially, to give support, answer questions, and reward the parent for the difficult task of learning a new way of interacting with the child. The consultant called the teacher every week to reward and support her for calling the parent. The consultant used peer group supervision to get *his* support for calling the teacher.

Prior to providing information or skill training, the consultant must do a thorough assessment of the problem. When the consultant has not yet gained sufficient conceptualization to propose an intervention or interventions at different levels, he/she has probably not yet asked enough questions. There is a tendency on the part of the consultant to feel pressure to respond to the needs of the consultee and to demonstrate competence. Caplan (1970) proposed that you demonstrate competence by the questions you ask, not by your answers. Not only are you modeling a problem-solving approach to the situation, but you are also increasing the likelihood that you will have sufficient information to make an informed judgment about an intervention.

Education as an intervention strategy has many advantages. It tends to be relatively nonthreatening to the consultees. Particularly in group formats in the form of workshops, the consultees do not demonstrate incompetence by admitting that there is a problem they do not know how to solve, as they often do when they approach a consultant for individual help. From the point of view of the consultant, the risk is low because people are unlikely to be upset. Education's primary disadvantage for the consultant is twofold: First, the payoffs may be relatively low. A variety of problems have to be addressed before competence is likely to be broad enough to handle a significant number of different *kinds* of problems. Even generalization from one client to the next is surprisingly low. One consultant found that it took 2 to 3 years before consultees were seeing similarities between types of problems presented that day and previous problems worked out successfully. The payoffs in terms of system change may be relatively low compared with the payoffs of some of the other intervention models, discussed later. The educational model requires that the problem be conceptualized as due to a lack of knowledge or skill. That level of intervention is not always appropriate. Finally, in systems that have large staff turnover, you are constantly training individuals who are then constantly leaving. No system change ever occurs, and the continued dependence of consultees on the consultant suggests that another intervention approach may be more appropriate.

The educational model assumes that the consultant has mental health information and skills. Some consultants seem to feel that knowledge of individual or group *process* is enough. Without specific psychological knowledge about the population served—whether children, criminals, the aged, parishioners, or special ethnic populations—the consultant quickly loses credibility. Knowledge and skills on the part of the consultant are necessary but not sufficient resources for effective consultation.

INDIVIDUAL-PROCESS MODEL

In the individual-process model, the consultant conceptualizes the difficulty on the part of the consultee in solving a community mental health-oriented problem as due primarily to the attitudes, motivation, intrapsychic conflicts, or personal style of the consultee. Intervention tends to be focused around eliminating defensive processes, resolving theme interferences, or facilitating personal growth. Typically the consultant has a dynamic or humanistic approach but may draw on other psychological theories.

The consultee-centered case consultation and the consultee-centered administrative consultation of Caplan (1970) follow this model. The consultee cannot solve the problems presented by the client because of over-involvement (one consultant had to deal with a teacher who decided to essentially adopt a child in her class), theme interference, lack of self-confidence, lack of objectivity, simple identification, transference, and characterological distortions. *Theme interference* is the most elaborately developed problem. It was defined by Caplan as a series of beliefs held by a person in which a particular situation characterizes an unsolved problem and leads inevitably to an unpleasant outcome.

Heller and Monahan, in their chapter on individual-process models, propose a useful reconceptualization of theme interference that allows them to intervene without the troublesome theoretical implications of unconscious motivation and the ethical problems of changing basic personality structure without the permission of the consultee. They propose that theme interferences are more usefully seen as stereotypes and, as stereotypes, are amenable to change.

One of the more common theme interferences that one consultant has found in the schools is that of teachers who discover incipient "homosexuals" in fourth- or fifth-grade classes (and who assume that being "homosexual" is a fate worse than death). A common dynamic found in this situation is an effeminate boy who is receiving significant peer group rejection for his sex-role-inappropriate behavior. By refocusing the problem on peer group rejection, by raising the issue of helping to move the child's behavior in a direction more acceptable to peers, and by providing alternative outcomes of effeminate behavior and homosexuality other than doom, the consultant can significantly reduce stereotypes about homosexuality and effeminate behavior. In contrast, as will be discussed later, a system-oriented person might raise questions about how to help the system become more accepting of a broader range of behaviors.

Individual-process consultation is strongly effective as an intervention depending on (1) how central the personality dynamic is for interfering with effective job functioning, (2) how often in the work situation client characteristics activate the consultee's interfering dynamics, (3) the centrality of the consultee in the system, and (4) staff turnover. At times an effective reduction in a theme interference (or stereotype) can be helpful for hundreds of clients served by that consultee. If police officers can change their basic stereotypes about an ethnic group that is common in the catchment area, the change in quality of service and quality of life in the area may be far reaching.

Systems Model

In the systems model, the consultant conceptualizes the difficulty on the part of the consultee in solving a community health-related problem as due primarily to the characteristics of the organization or community to which the client and consultee belong. Intervention is focused around changing channels of communication, power, support, and influence. Typically such a consultant has a systems or organizational development approach but may draw on interpersonal theories of psychology.

The systems model is foreign to many mental health consultants, although more and more are training primarily at this level. For the traditionally trained mental health professional who is moving into consultation for the first time, the terminology of the systems model is likely to be new. In order to be responsive to this problem, Schmuck, in his chapter on system orientations, has been careful to provide definitions of the basic assumptions and terms. It would well serve the community mental health consultant to study these terms and be sure that the basic conceptualizations are understood before doing consultation.

Knowledge about system dynamics plays a major role in the day-to-day life of the consultant. The consultant who does not recognize what role the system plays in fostering and maintaining pathology will be forever confused as to why particular patterns of problems exist or why various attempts to solve systemic problems at the individual level are unsuccessful.

There is little relationship between the systems approach and Caplan's administrative consultation since Caplan (1970) referred to program planning, not system intervention. It is not necessary to use the language of the systems theorists or organizational development people to think in terms of community organization; for example, several parents at an elementary school asked teachers for help in a problem in which fourth-grade boys and girls were kissing and petting. The teachers suggested that the parents meet with the community mental consultant assigned to the school. In the evening meeting, the parents described a pattern of behavior in which the boys and girls in the fourth grade were meeting inside the only theater in town, waiting until the cartoon was over, and then madly grabbing and kissing each other. A boy who refused to kiss a girl was threatened. Several system characteristics contributed to this problem. First, the school district had formed a middle school the previous year, and the fifth grades had transferred to that school. Second, the sixth-graders had traditionally been the troublemakers in the school. The fourth-graders had been very quiet. Third, the town was small, with no recreational centers or programs, and the single theater was the social gathering place of the community. The consultant first discussed with the parents the delight that children of middle and late elementary school age have in being involved in forbidden behavior. The ritualistic patterns suggested that hormones had little to do with the "sexual" behavior. When the parents looked at the behavior as preadolescent exploring of forbidden behavior, they were able to relax considerably. The discussion then led to the problem of boredom as a precursor to socially inappropriate behaviors in children. That discussion led to the lack of recreational opportunities. The parents then began plans to contact local churches to see if they could develop a recreation center for kids of all ages. An individual-education approach could have led to disciplinary approaches, and an individual-process approach could have focused on the sexuality concerns in parents; a systems orientation led to treating the problem at the community level.

System intervention is likely to be somewhat riskier in terms of payoff, since systems, by definition, are complex and difficult to change. Indeed the maintenance aspects of systems works toward ensuring that change does *not* occur. When a systemwide intervention does occur, the impact can be impressive. Not only have the clients benefitted, but because of the maintenance aspects of systems, the changes tend to become independent of the people who occupy positions within the system and thus, regardless of consultee turnover, the changes are likely to be relatively enduring.

Most mental health consultation models have focused on one or another levels of analysis to the exclusion of others. Ultimately consultational intervention must be seen not as theory-based, but rather as process; and the approach to specific problems should be seen as an exercise in multiple-theory application. A consultant who values the interaction between models may view a problem from a number of different perspectives with the advantage of gaining additional information and ultimately more alternatives for intervention strategies.

A broad problem-solving approach includes

1. Those theories that focus primarily on the intrapsychic or inner-life environment

2. Those theories that focus primarily on the ecological environment

3. Those theories that focus primarily on the psychosocial or psycho-ecological setting

4. Those theories that focus primarily on systems

Theories subsumed under (1) probably characterize a major portion of the training received by mental health consultants, and are thus familiar to most, if not all, consultants who received formal training in a clinical context. The difficulty with this backdrop is that the emphasis of psychology has been on variations in an individual's behavior, an emphasis that somehow inhibits the consultant in escaping this pervasive force so that he/she may conceptualize problems at other levels. Each level can contribute to problem conceptualization, and wherever possible, each level should be utilized.

The unique position of the community mental health consultant provides a perspective on the system generally unavailable to anyone in the system itself. The consultant also has the mobility to interact with aspects of the system in a way unavailable to the members. It is not unusual that a problem can be conceptualized at all three levels of intervention. The consultant has to make a decision about the most effective strategy. Where does the system give permission for intervention? Some questions raised by each model include these: Is the system ready for more involved interventions? What would be the impact on the system of interventions at each of the levels? What are the risks and probable payoffs? How much energy is required, given the benefits of solving this problem, at different levels or even at all? What are the ethical problems raised by intervention at each level?

REFERENCES

Blake, R. R., & Mouton, J. S. *Consultation.* Reading, Mass.: Addison-Wesley, 1976.

Caplan, G. *The theory and practice of mental health consultation.* New York: Basic Books, 1970.

Chapter 3

MENTAL HEALTH CONSULTATION
An Educational Approach

Timothy G. Kuehnel, Ph.D.
Julie M. Kuehnel, Ph.D.

An educational approach to mental health consultation conceptualizes the difficulty on the part of the consultee in solving a mental health-related problem as due primarily to a lack of skill or knowledge. Although most consultants who use this approach have a behavior modification orientation, the strategy to be presented may be used by consultants espousing other orientations, such as client-centered, rational-emotive, process, or dynamic approaches. That is, the educational process of consultation may be adapted to impart a variety of content to consultees. The focus of this chapter is on the process of educational mental health consultation, which involves *behavioral* approaches including assessing presenting problems, imparting information, and actively teaching skills to a consultee through the use of instructions, modeling, shaping, behavioral rehearsal with structured feedback, and homework assignments. This emphasis includes the consultant's provision of relevant mental health information or knowledge to the consultee. This chapter does not focus on the content of such information since acquisition of this content is central to the consultant's professional education. Development of expertise as a consultant requires knowledge of that content. The practice of mental health consultation using an educational model requires an understanding of how that knowledge or skill is transferred to the consultee.

The overall goal of an educational approach to consultation is to change the consultee's behavior in handling a particular client problem or problem situation in the work environment. In this way, educational consultation does not differ significantly from other consultative approaches.

The differences between this and other approaches arise in the assumptions that are made regarding how this goal is attained.

According to Caplan (1970), there are four possible reasons the consultee may be having difficulty: lack of knowledge, lack of skill, lack of self-confidence, and lack of professional objectivity. The educational model focuses on the first two of these dimensions and assumes changes in these dimensions will often lead to changes in the latter two.

The assumption is made that changing the consultee's knowledge and behavior in dealing with a problem client or situation will result in a change in the consultee's attitude or perceptions of the problem. Many consultative approaches assume that the consultee must first experience a change in his/her perception of a work-related problem and that this alteration in perception will affect the consultee's behavior. These changes are then assumed to affect client behavior and to be generalized by the consultee to future problems (Alpert, 1976). As Mannino and Shore (1970, 1975) pointed out, there is little direct evidence or systematic research to support this chain of assumptions. An educational approach is based upon actively targeting problem behaviors, training the consultee in alternative methods of handling the problem behaviors, and helping the consultee to implement programs and monitor client progress. This training, or educational strategy in consultation assumes that perceptions will change as a result of this process and is equally tenable to the proposition that changes in perception must precede changes in behavior.

An educational model of consultation assumes that (1) behavior is learned and is related to the social environment of the consultee and client, (2) the social environment provides cues for behavior and reinforces or punishes that behavior, and (3) in order for meaningful changes in the social system, the consultee, or the client to occur, changes in behavioral contingencies must occur.

The content or focus of an educational approach to consultation are typically derived from the theory and practice of behavior modification (Bandura, 1969). Applications of educational consultation have included providing teachers and counselors with general instruction in behavior modification principles (McKeown, Henry, & Forehand, 1975), contingency management (Ayllon & Roberts, 1974), feedback and praise (Cossairt, Hall, & Hopkins, 1973), and positive practice techniques (Azrin & Powers, 1975). Other consultants have helped teachers set up token economies (Ayllon, Layman, & Kandel, 1975) and provided teachers with comprehensive classroom management packages (Jones & Eimers, 1975). Similar applications of behavioral principles have been used by consultants working with business and industry (Brown & Presbie, 1976) and on such problems as institutional change in social service settings (Reppucci &

Saunders, 1974), staff performance (Patterson, Griffin, & Panyan, 1976), supervision behavior (Goldstein & Sorcher, 1973), and staff management (Quilitch, 1975).

These and similar studies provided some indication of the *content* utility of these behavioral interventions, but less attention has been paid to the consulting *process* necessary to provide consultees with the knowledge and skill necessary to implement and maintain such programs. Nietzel, Winett, MacDonald, and Davidson (1977) noted that most behavioral intervention programs terminate on dates that correspond closely to the appearance of a publication describing the project's "initial" results. This is despite the popular portrayal of these behavioral principles and procedures as being transmitted quickly and learned easily. Hersen and Bellack (1978), Graziano (1969), and Reppucci and Saunders (1974) also noted that many behavioral consultants have failed in their attempts to help consultees implement behavioral programs. Failure can often be traced to institutional constraints, staff resistance, a lack of administrative support, political realities, language problems, and a variety of other factors. Apparently additional attention must be devoted by behavioral consultants to the process used to provide the consultee with the requisite knowledge and skill necessary to carry out these interventions and to issues that will facilitate their implementation and maintenance.

Other behavioral consultation approaches focus heavily on the *client* behaviors to be changed through the use of behavioral approaches (Jason and Ferone, 1978) or on the consultee's and consultant's behavior in eliciting information about problems and developing plans to deal with the situation (Bergan, 1977). The process to be described here has as its primary focus changing *consultee* behaviors. This chapter describes and illustrates with examples the *process* of educational consultation as the consultant proceeds through five phases of consultation.

The first is *entry and goal setting,* during which the consultant and consultee or consultee organization arrive at a contract specifying the parameters of the relationship and the roles and responsibilities of the consultant and consultee, set the goals of the consultation, and establish a mechanism and criteria for evaluating the progress of the consultation. The second phase is *problem specification.* The consultant helps the consultee to specify the problem in terms of behavioral excesses and deficits exhibited by the client (or system), to determine the client's strengths and assets that may be brought to bear on the problem, to target specific client behaviors to be changed, and to collect baseline data on these target behaviors. The third phase is *knowledge and skill acquisition.* Through the use of structured role playing, feedback, modeling, coaching, and prompting, the consultant trains the consultee in alternative strategies and behaviors to remedy the problem. The consultant also provides information relevant to the consultee's understanding of the problem. The fourth phase is *implementation and evaluation*. The consultant helps the consultee implement alternative strategies for dealing with the problem situation and evaluates their effectiveness. In the course of consultation, these phases may overlap and are recycled through as the problem becomes clearer or shifts in focus. The final phase to be discussed is *termination* of the consultation relationship. This phase includes emphasis on maintenance and generalization of the knowledge and skill acquired during consultation. Potential problems the consultant may encounter and some guidelines for overcoming these problems are included in each of these phases.

ENTRY AND GOAL SETTING

The first phase in educational consultation, as in other forms of consultation, is entry and goal setting. Unfortunately most writers in this field concentrate on the results of their behaviorally oriented consulting efforts, leaving the details of this crucial phase to the reader's imagination (Dorr, 1977, Reppucci, 1977).

Levine (1973) and Sarason, Levine, Goldenberg, Cherlin, and Bennet (1968) noted that there is a period of time during the initial stages of consultation when the consultee(s) are testing the newcomer in various ways. The consultee is seeking answers to the following types of questions about the consultant: What does he/she want? Whose side is she/he on? Is the consultant competent? What will he/she do for me? As Reppucci (1977) noted, this phase must be successfully negotiated if a productive intervention is to occur. The educationally oriented consultant must recognize and tailor the focus and pace of the consultation to the norms of behavior and interaction of the existing institutional staff. Rather than expecting an open-armed reception to which a prepackaged and validated solution can be applied, the educational consultant must establish rapport and gain the sanction and consent of all parties relevant to the consultation effort. It should be noted that educational consultation may be distinguished from education in that (1) the consultee is relatively free to accept or reject the suggestions for change made by the consultant and (2) although the process of educational consultation remains constant, there is not an a priori planned curriculum. The purpose of this phase is to establish a climate for working with the consultee based upon his/her needs and desires. The following steps need to occur in this phase.

First, the consultant must begin the process of identifying and defining the roles and responsibilities of the consultant and the consultee. Typically the educational consultant assumes an indirect relationship to the client and works directly with the consultee, who retains responsibility for implementing changes in line with the goals of the consultation. The consultant will typically identify the following things in specific terms: (1) those areas of psychological knowledge that the consultant can make available to the consultee are identified; (2) the strategies for learning, training, or problem solving that will be used are determined; (3) issues with respect to confidentiality are noted; (4) the person(s) to whom the consultant is responsible is specified; and (5) the where and when of potential interaction are provided.

Educational consultants do not attempt to communicate all this information in didactic terms. Rather they provide a brief overview of these areas and then demonstrate with a potential consultee the process they would use to assist the consultee in skillfully utilizing one of the knowledge areas germane to a suggested problem. The demonstration involves targeting of problem behaviors, modeling, and behavior rehearsal as an appropriate solution is shaped, since this is the process used in educational consultation. The purpose of the demonstration is not to make the consultee proficient in the use of a particular behavioral intervention but rather to illustrate potential problem foci and the consultation process that may be used. Our experience has been that this demonstration generates enthusiasm and is often the beginning of a congenial relationship between the consultant and the consultee. This is in striking contrast to the anxiety and reserve that often accompany traditional entry strategies as consultants attempt to explain how they might be of assistance (Smith, 1975). The demonstration models more than the use of a "bag of tricks" that can be employed by the consultees. Potential consultees have a firsthand opportunity to observe the consultant's openness, warmth, listening skills, and facility in defining problems and in so doing build rapport with the consultant. The consultant can also use this demonstration as an opportunity to begin stressing implementation, by asking such questions as "How could you make use of these or similar techniques in your work situation?"

At this point, the consultant asks for the consultees' sanction and consent to continue. Negative stereotypes about who the consultant is and what the consultant does have been reduced, and the consultees can make a more informed decision about whether or not they want to continue with the consultant and the consultation.

An educationally oriented consultant is likely, through a series of questions, to define in behavioral terms those aspects of the consultative relationship that will engender cooperation. The consultant might ask for the following events to occur: "Would you be willing to meet with me on Thursday from 3 P.M. to 4 P.M. to work on defining the problems you are faced with? Would you be willing to practice with me some alternative ways of dealing with these problems? Would you be willing to have me observe your handling of these problems? Would you be willing to have me observe your handling of these problems in your work setting so that we might determine the refinements that need to be made and future directions in which we may want to move? Would you be willing to try the solutions we develop in your work situation? Etc.'' When the consultee answers questions similar to these, the consultant has defined this portion of the consulting relationship. The consultant must also contract with the consultee as to his/her cooperative behavior. Agreements typically revolve around issues such as spending a specific amount of time with the consultee, engaging in participative problem identification, developing intervention strategies, and providing useful feedback to the consultee on improvements observed and progress made. In addition, the consultant should negotiate an agreement for the general content and focus of the consultation (i.e., ''dealing with student management problems'' or ''improving interstaff communication skills'' or ''facilitating interagency cooperation''). These agreements and the answers to the other questions can then be transformed into a written letter of agreement so that all parties are clear regarding their behavioral commitment during the consultation and the general content and goals of the arrangements made.

PROBLEM SPECIFICATION

The second phase of behavioral consultation is problem identification and specification. The importance of this phase is highlighted by a recent study of consultant skills and of the implementation and outcome of consultation. Bergan and Tombari (1975) found that, once consultative problem solving was effectively carried through the problem identification phase, problem solution almost invariably resulted. When the consultant lacked skill in problem identification or was inefficient in this phase, there was a substantial likelihood that problem solving would never be initiated.

During this phase of educational consultation, the consultant determines the consultee's concern and helps the consultee specify the client's behavioral excesses and deficits. By focusing on behaviors to be changed, the consultee's perception of the problem is shifted from a global, anxiety-producing set, such as ''he's a bad kid; he's too aggressive,'' to a more balanced perception, such as ''we need to help him alter some of his excess hitting behaviors by teaching him some appropriate ways of gaining the attention that he wants.'' This ''reframing'' of the problem makes it seem more manageable to the consultee and focuses energy toward solving the problem rather than dwelling on its past difficulty or simply labeling it.

The consultant then helps the consultee determine the client's assets and strengths so that these may be used in programs to alter the client's behavior. What does the client do particularly well or has he/she done well in the past? What interpersonal resources (e.g., another teacher with whom the client gets along well, cooperative and concerned parents, certain friends in class) does the client have that can be brought to bear on the problem.

The third step is to help the consultee place this information into a more global picture by making a functional analysis of the problem. The type of questions to be answered here are these: Who reinforces the client with sympathy and attention or emotional reactions? What reinforcers will the client gain or lose if the problem behaviors are removed? The consultee is then helped to select one or two client behaviors on which to begin working. When there are multiple problem behaviors, the consultant can help the consultee choose those behaviors to begin working on that are more likely to respond positively and/or are likely to influence other behaviors in a positive direction. Beginning with smaller, more easily manageable behaviors achieves several purposes. First, since the consultee will be learning and practicing *new* skills, it is easier to learn on simpler behaviors. Second, by beginning small, the consultee is more likely to experience success, which will provide motivation, confidence, and positive expectations when beginning to work on more difficult or complex problem behaviors. Consultees, like clients, learn new behaviors best in small, manageable steps.

When one or two target behaviors have been specified, the consultee is given instructions for collecting simple baseline data in order to ascertain the severity of the problem and to provide a data base for evaluating the effectiveness of an intervention. Simple frequency counts are usually sufficient. If the target behaviors are high in frequency (occur constantly throughout the day), a time-sampling procedure (i.e., recording the frequency for two half-hour periods per day) is suggested. In this way data gathering is not so burdensome that the consultee refuses to do it. It also does not require more data than are necessary to evaluate the effectiveness of the intervention.

In setting goals with the consultee, it is important for the consultant to distinguish between first-order and second-order change (Watzlawik, Weakland, & Fisch, 1974). According to this formulation, first-order change occurs when a problem has been misconceptualized from the outset so that interventions are based on inappropriate assumptions. In the school setting, for example, it would be erroneous to assume that the model student was "one who stays glued to his seat and desk all day, continually looks at his teacher or his text/workbook, does not talk [to] or in fact look at other children, does not talk unless asked by the teacher, hopefully does not laugh or sing (or at the wrong time) and assuredly passes silently in halls'' (Winnet & Winkler, 1972, p. 501). Such an assumption may lead to a highly conforming, but perhaps rigid and nonspontaneous child. In this example, the educational consultant who worked with the consultee to define goals in line with this description would be engaging in first-order change. It is, therefore, the ethical obligation of the consultant to examine the aims and potential impact of their consultation efforts and not aid consultees in attainment of inappropriate goals (Emery & Marholin, 1977).

KNOWLEDGE AND SKILL ACQUISITION

Once the consultee has specified the problem in behavioral terms and collected some baseline data, the knowledge and skill acquisition phase of the consultation process begins. The heart of this phase of educational consultation is provision of relevant information in understandable terms and structured role playing with feedback. That is, once the consultee has a cursory understanding of the relevant mental health principles involved, he/she learns new skills and alternative methods of handling a problem situation by trying them out during the individual or group consultation session. This approach to knowledge and skill acquisition is similar to the microteaching approach developed by Emmer and Millett (1970), the microconsultation format developed by Goodwin, Garvey, and Barclay (1971), and the social skills training program of Liberman, King, and DeRisi (1975). These methods were developed in response to findings that learning without experiencing how something works is usually not sufficient to produce lasting systematic changes in behavior.

Although this process can be carried out on an individual basis with a consultee, a group consultation format is particularly helpful during this phase since it provides for multiple sources of feedback and multiple models and alternatives for dealing with a specific problem. Often feedback and modeling by peers regarding the handling of a particular situation are more powerful than feedback and modeling by the consultant alone. The group format also offers many more sources of reinforcement for consultees as they try new skills and new solutions to problems that they have been experiencing. This peer reinforcement of efforts and learning of new skills builds a reinforcing network into the group that may be maintained in their everyday working environment. As consultees begin to implement the skills that have been learned in the consultation group, their successes are ''public'' and can lead to positive expectations on the part of the other group members regarding the usefulness and applicability of the techniques. These positive expectations provide motivation for continued effort on the part of consultees whose problems are worked on in other sessions, and consultees come to feel comfortable in trying new techniques because of the support that the group provides.

The training phase begins with the consultant engaging the consultee in a dry run. The consultant asks the consultee to describe the most recent occurrence of the problem. The consultant then simulates the scene in the session by using simple props, and the consultant or another group member takes the role of the client. The consultee demonstrates how he/she usually handles the situation. The consultee's behavioral excesses and deficiencies and level of skill are usually readily apparent to the consultant as well as to the consultee.

At the end of the dry run, the consultant provides specific feedback to the consultee. The consultant begins with positive feedback and solicits positive feedback from the group on the consultee's handling of the problem before making specific suggestions for improvement.

To be most effective, feedback and suggestions for change to the consultee must *describe* what it is that the consultee did or did not do. In the case of the consultee who is working on a student's problem of acting out in class, a positive comment might be that she/he was quick to recognize the source of the problem and attempted to intervene quickly. Suggestions are also stated in specific behavioral terms, for example, "rather than shouting at the student across the room, it would be more effective if you walked over, got within 3 feet of her, and made your comment in a low tone that only she could hear." Specific descriptive feedback and suggestions for change are more effective in facilitating the consultee's learning than general feedback such as "You certainly let her know what was on your mind, but this time make it more personal." In this latter instance, consultees are left with some vague notion that they can improve, but there is no clear indication of the specific behaviors they engaged in that the observers favored and no information about what they must do in order to be more personal. When feedback and suggestions for change are described in terms of behaviors to be changed, the consultees know exactly what they can do to improve the interaction.

A second consideration in giving feedback and suggestions for change following a dry run is that the consultant should adopt a shaping attitude. Negative feedback should be stated as suggestions for change and should be limited to one or two behaviors to be tried in the next rehearsal. The consultant should not bombard the consultee with a whole list of suggestions for change that are likely to make the consultee feel inadequate and overload his/her ability to assimilate the information. Once the consultee has gone through a dry run and received positive feedback and suggestions from the rest of the group and the consultant, the consultee engages in a behavioral rehearsal. This means that the consultant sets up the situation again and asks the consultee to rehearse the interaction with the "client" while incorporating the one or two suggestions for improvement that were made during the feedback session. It is important to keep these rehearsals crisp and short (i.e., 1 to 2 min.). At the end of the behavioral rehearsal is another feedback session. At this point it may be very helpful for the consultant or another member of the group to model some alternative ways the consultee may handle the situation in the future. By having someone demonstrate an alternative way to handle the situation, the consultee may be able to assimilate more information on how to handle the situation than she/he may through instruction and suggestions alone. Once consultees have observed a demonstration of how the situation might be handled, they engage in another behavioral rehearsal incorporating those elements of the demonstration that they felt would be helpful. If the consultee is having trouble engaging in some of the suggested behaviors or using some of the behaviors from the demonstration, the consultant might coach or prompt the consultee during the behavioral rehearsal. The consultant may use hand signals to prompt the consultee to smile or not to smile during a particular interaction or to maintain eye contact with the "client" during the rehearsal. Pointing to the ear may indicate the need to speak up; to the mouth, to smile. Prompting and coaching provide direction and support for the consultee to practice the new behaviors and increase likelihood that the consultee will experience success during the behavioral rehearsal. It is important to build in as much success as possible for the consultee during the training session in order to increase motivation and improve the consultee's self-confidence in handling the situation. Behavioral rehearsal is engaged in until the consultee reaches a criterion level of performance.

This process is useful in training consultees in a wide variety of interpersonal skills. A consultee may be having difficulty giving effective negative feedback to a subordinate or supervisee. Helping the consultee acquire the appropriate nonverbal and verbal communication skills necessary to provide feedback that is specific, to the point, and more effective may be the content of several consultation sessions. The educational consultation process remains the same. The consultant initially engages the consultee in a dry run to demonstrate how he/she normally interacts or gives feedback to the particular subordinate. The consultant then gives feedback regarding the positive aspects of his/her performance along with suggestions for change. Modeling, prompting, and coaching are effective tools for helping the consultee change his/her handling of the situation. The consultee then rehearses alternative skills or behaviors until the consultee demonstrates mastery of at least one or two of the skills necessary to implement a solution. Always end on a successful rehearsal rather than pushing the consultee by adding suggestions until they fail. Consultees learn better through a *series* of small successes.

IMPLEMENTATION AND EVALUATION

After the immediate objective of effecting change in the *knowledge and skill* of the consultee has been attained, the consultant and consultee may begin the implementation phase. Since the ultimate goal is to bring about positive change in the consultee's client group, this phase is very important. Based on their review of those few studies that have directly and systematically attempted to investigate variables that influence generalization of behavioral changes from therapy to natural settings, Koegel and Rincover (1977) concluded that generalization does not occur without special intervention and attention to this process. Similarly, if the consultant does not program for this occurrence, the consultees will frequently become frustrated by their inability to apply their new knowledge and skill consistently and effectively.

The consultant may begin phasing in implementation by giving the consultee a "homework assignment." The consultant may ask the consultee to try out the behaviors that have been learned during the training sessions in the real-life problem situations. The decision to give the consultee a homework assignment is based on several criteria. First, has the consultee learned the behaviors well enough that he/she is likely to experience success in carrying them out in a real-life situation? It is important not to send a consultee back to handle a real-life situation before he/she has learned the necessary skills. An alternative is to adopt a shaping attitude and give the consultee a homework assignment that does not involve him/her directly in the presenting problem situation. In the case of a problem student, the teacher may have practiced some skills in giving praise and mild social punishment, but in the consultant's opinion he/she is not yet skilled enough in the use of this and other methods to tackle the presenting problem. Consequently the consultant may give a homework assignment that has the consultee practice the new skills with more manageable children in his or her class; "The next time another child is starting to act up in class, I want you to use the mild social punishment skills we practiced today; that is, move within 3 feet of that child, get eye contact with that child, and, using a low tone, tell the child to stop the particular behavior that you want stopped."

In the case of a consultee learning to give more effective feedback to a subordinate, the homework assignment may be to "choose a supervisee with whom you have a strong relationship, and during your next session with him or her on Tuesday morning, use the feedback skills we have practiced today [make eye contact, *describe* the behaviors you like and those that need improvement, and solicit her/his reaction]. Let me know how it went in our next session.'' Giving homework assignments that do not involve the consultee with the primary problem gives the consultee a chance to practice the skills learned in the training session in the real-life environment. It also provides an opportunity for the consultee to overlearn those skills and experience some success in using them so that they become a natural part of his/her behavioral repertoire.

At the beginning of the next session, the consultant should check on how the homework assignment went, an activity that reinforces the consultee's efforts to carry it out. It is important to check on how the homework assignment went in order to set the agenda for the training session. If the consultee completed the assignment successfully, the consultant increases the complexity of the skills to be learned or adds more behaviors for the consultee to learn. If the consultee did not attempt to carry out the homework assignment, several things should be considered. First, the consultant must consider whether the homework assignment was too difficult. If this is the case, the consultant may engage the consultee in more rehearsal of the skills involved and give the homework assignment again or give a simpler assignment. Second, the consultant needs to build in some reinforcers for the consultee to try out the homework assignments in a real-life environment. A very powerful reinforcer, particularly in group consultation, is the time and attention given to the consultee by the consultant and the other group members for completing or not completing homework assignments. Very often a lot of time and attention is spent discussing why the consultee did not carry out the homework assignment. This time allocation is the reverse of what should happen.

In group consultation, time and attention should be devoted to those who made an effort to complete their homework assignments. Another way of facilitating homework completion is for the consultant to stop by or telephone and prompt the consultee regarding the homework assignment. This may be as simple as asking the consultee how it is going during the week and whether he or she has tried the skills practiced during training, and reinforcing the consultee's efforts. As the consultee becomes more skilled, the consultant increases the emphasis on implementation with the presenting problem. Homework assignments can become more complex, and monitoring of their effectiveness may involve observations of the consultee in his or her natural environment in order to add refinements to the consultant's skills. In addition, the data that the consultee is collecting are continuously assessed in order to provide continuous feedback to the consultee and consultant on the effectiveness of the intervention.

As the consultation progresses, the consultant and the consultee need to review the goals set initially. As goals are attained, new goals may be negotiated or a decision may be made to terminate the consultation.

TERMINATION

The ending phase of educational consultation has many of the same elements as the termination of any other form of consultation. Methods for dealing with termination should include the use of time structure, fading procedures, reinforcement of consultee gains, and planning for the future.

A definite time structure assists the termination process in two ways. First, the time structure that was developed in the entry and goal-setting phase will help the consultee to anticipate the ending point. Time limits and target dates often assist in motivating the consultee to use the time available wisely and to implement newly acquired skills with her or his clients while the consultant's support and troubleshooting assistance are readily accessible. Attainment of the goals set during this initial phase provides a mutually agreed upon indication that the consultation has achieved its purpose.

As the end of the consultation nears, the consultation meetings can be shortened and scheduled at longer intervals. This procedure is known as *fading* and makes the consultee less and less dependent on the consultant's advice and approval. After meeting with a consultee for 2 hrs per week for 6 weeks, the meeting might be scheduled for 30 min. semiweekly. When the sessions are spaced further apart, newly acquired skills and knowledge can be practiced and independently sustained by the consultee for longer and longer periods of time. The available evidence indicates that behavioral changes are not maintained if training is terminated abruptly (Walker, Mattson, & Buckley, 1971; Friedlander, 1968). Therefore educational consultation that focuses on increasing consultee skills needs to incorporate a fading process to increase the likelihood of skill maintenance.

Even with a time-limited and goal-oriented approach to consultation such as this, the consultee often fails to internalize achievements and depends heavily on the consultant for reinforcement. Since gains typically occur in small increments, it is helpful for the educational consultant to review periodically with the consultee the overall progress that has been made and to have the consultee gradually assume responsibility for observing and reinforcing himself or herself for these gains. If a group consultation approach has been utilized, the consultant can promote the reinforcing power of the consultee's colleagues upon the individual gains of consultees. This may facilitate a reinforcing network within the consultee agency that will continue after the formal consultation has ended. There is some evidence that suggests that the existence of a ''core'' group within the consultee's organization that supports the consultee's efforts and progress and assists in troubleshooting difficulties enhances the likelihood of the consultee's continued use of the skills acquired and the interventions that have been implemented (Fairweather, Sanders, & Tornatzky, 1974). If a group consultation approach has been utilized, the consultant might suggest that this group continue to meet at regular intervals in order to serve this purpose. If the consultation was with an individual, the consultant might assist the consultee in identifying and establishing a group from which he or she could receive support and assistance.

Another important aspect of the termination is helping the consultee plan for the future. This can be facilitated by periodically highlighting the problem-solving process utilized by the consultant. That is, the consultee has learned to identify problems in behavioral terms, to collect baseline data, to specify small and easily attainable goals, to practice alternative solutions to the identified problem, to implement solutions, and to monitor progress. These skills can be used by the consultee to handle similar future concerns.

ADVANTAGES AND DISADVANTAGES OF AN EDUCATIONAL APPROACH TO MENTAL HEALTH CONSULTATION

The educational approach offers mental health consultants several advantages over more traditional types of consultation. First, the methods are suited to the time constraints often found in community settings. The goals of educational consultation are to bring about limited, functional changes. Second, the educational consultant conceptualizes problems as arising from an interaction between the client and his/her environment rather than as being intrinsic to the person. In this way there is a congruence with the emphasis in community psychology on changing the client's social environment or increasing the client's skills in coping with the environment. Third, educational consultation procedures are sufficiently concrete and operationalized to be quickly learned by student consultants. They can be disseminated conveniently when found effective. Thus educational consultation can be viewed as potentially adding some working muscles to the philosophical skeleton of community mental health, community psychology, and community psychiatry (Liberman & Bryan, 1977; Mannino & Shore, 1971). In addition, the empirical orientation basic to the type of educational consultation elaborated on here facilitates evaluation. Because specification and measurement are intrinsic to a behavioral approach, evaluation of consultation outcome is a natural by-product. Evaluation promotes an evolutionary development of procedures that are refined or discarded by the consultant and consultee as experience dictates.

One initial disadvantage of the educational consultation model is that the procedures and processes involved are different from what consultees have often come to expect from consultants. Potential consultees are more used to the idea of simply talking about their problems with a consultant rather than actively playing roles and learning new skills. Initially there may be some resistance to this more active approach. In the course of discussing educational consultation, we have tried to include some suggestions for overcoming these resistances as they arise. We hope these suggestions will be helpful to a consultant initiating this mode of consultation in an organization. We have found that, once consultees have had experience with this model, they are enthusiastic and responsive.

References

Alpert, J. L. Conceptual bases of mental health consultation. *Professional Psychology,* 1976, *7,* 619-626.

Ayllon, T., Layman, D., & Kandel, H. J. A behavioral educational alternative to drug control of hyperactive children. *Journal of Applied Behavior Analysis,* 1975, *8,* 137-146.

———, & Roberts, M. Eliminating discipline problems by strengthening academic performance. *Journal of Applied Behavior Analysis,* 1974, *7,* 71-76.

Azrin, H. H., & Powers, M. A. Eliminating classroom disturbances of emotionally disturbed children by positive practice procedure. *Behavior Therapy,* 1975, *6,* 525-534.

Bandura, A. *Principles of behavior modification.* New York: Holt, Rinehart & Winston, 1969.

Bergen, J., & Tombari, M. The analysis of verbal interactions occurring during consultation. *Journal of School Psychology,* 1975, *13,* 209–227.

Bergan, J. R. *Behavioral consultation.* Columbus, Ohio: Merrill, 1977.

Brown, P. L., & Presbie, R. J. *Behavior modification in business, industry and government.* New Paltz, N.Y.: Behavior Improvement Associates, 1976.

Caplan, G. *The theory and practice of mental health consultation.* New York: Basic Books, 1970.

Cossairt, A., Hall, R. V., & Hopkins, B. L. The effects of experimenter instructions, feedback, and praise on teacher praise and student attending behavior. *Journal of Applied Behavior Analysis,* 1973, *6,* 89-100.

Dorr, D. Some practical suggestions on behavioral consultation with teachers. *Professional Psychology,* 1977, *8,* 95-102.

Emery, R. E., & Marholin, D. An applied behavior analysis of delinquency: The irrelevancy of relevant behavior. *American Psychologist,* 1977, *32,* 860-873.

Emmer, E., & Millett, G. *Improving teaching through experimentation,* New York: Holt, Rinehart & Winston, 1970.

Fairweather, G. W., Sanders, D. H., & Tornatzky, L. G. *Creating change in mental health organizations.* Elmsford, N.Y.: Pergamon Press, 1974.

Friedlander, F. A comparative study of consulting processes and group development. *Journal of Applied Behavioral Science,* 1968, *4,* 377-399.

Goldstein, A. P., & Sorcher, M. Changing managerial behavior by applied learning techniques. *Training and Development Journal,* 1973, *27,* 36-39.

Goodwin, D. L., Garvey, W. P., & Barclay, J. R. Microconsultation and behavior analysis: A method of training psychologists as behavioral consultants. *Journal of Consulting and Clinical Psychology,* 1971, *37,* 355-363.

Graziano, A. M. Clinical innovation and the mental health power structure: A social case history. *American Psychologist,* 1969, *24,* 10-18.

Hersen, M., & Bellack, A. S. Staff training and consultation. In M. Hersen & A. S. Bellack (Eds.), *Behavior therapy in the psychiatric setting.* Baltimore: Williams & Wilkins, 1978.

Jason, L. A., & Ferone, L. Behavioral versus process consultation interventions in school settings. *American Journal of Community Psychology,* 1978, *6,* 531-543.

Jones, F. H., & Eimers, R. C. Role playing to train elementary teachers to use classroom management "Skill Package." *Journal of Applied Behavior Analysis,* 1975, *8,* 421-433.

Koegel, R. L., & Rincover, A. Research on the difference between generalization and maintenance in extra-therapy responding. *Journal of Applied Behavior Analysis,* 1977, *10,* 1-12.

Levine, M. Problems of entry in light of some postulates of practice in community psychology. In I. I. Goldenberg (Ed.), *The helping professions in the world of action.* Lexington, Mass.: Heath, 1973.

Liberman, R. P., & Bryan, E. Behavior therapy in a community mental health center. *American Journal of Psychiatry,* 1977, *134,* 401-406.

_____, King, L.W., & DeRisi, W.J. *Personal effectiveness: Guiding people to assert their feelings & improve their social skills.* Champagne, Ill., Research Press, 1975.

Mannino, F. & Shore, M. *Consultation research in mental health and related fields: A critical review of the literature.* Washington, D.C.: U.S. Department of Health, Education, & Welfare, PHS Pub #2122, 1971.

_____, & _____. The effects of consultation: A review of empirical studies. *American Journal of Community Psychology,* 1975, *3,* 1-21.

McKeown, D., Jr., Henry, E. A., & Forehand, R. Generalization to the classroom of principles of behavior modification taught to teachers. *Behavior Research and Therapy,* 1975, *13,* 85-92.

Nietzel, M. T., Winett, R. A., MacDonald, M. L., & Davidson, W. S. *Behavioral approaches to community psychology.* Elmsford, N.Y.: Pergamon Press, 1977.

Patterson, E. T., Griffin, J. C., & Panyan, M. C. Incentive maintenance of self-help skill training programs for non-professional personnel. *Journal of Behavior Therapy and Experimental Psychiatry,* 1976, *7,* 249-253.

Quilitch, H. R. A comparison of three staff-management procedures. *Journal of Applied Behavior Analysis,* 1975, *8,* 59-66.

Randolph, D. L. Behavioral consultation as a means of improving the quality of a counseling program. *The School Counselor,* 1972, *20,30-35.*

Reppucci, N. D. Implementation issues for the behavior modifier as institutional change agent. *Behavior Therapy,* 1977, *8,* 594-605.

_____, & Saunders, J.T. Social psychology of behavior modification: Problems of implementation in natural settings. *American Psychologist,* 1974, *29,* 649-660.

Sarason, S. B., Levine, M., Goldenberg, I. I., Cherlin, D. K., & Bennet, E. M. *Psychology in the community settings.* New York: Wiley, 1966.

Smith, B. L. Assertion training as an entry strategy for consultation with school administrators. *The Counseling Psychologist,* 1975, *5,* 79-84.

Walker, H. M., Mattson, R. H., & Buckley, N. K. The functional analysis of behavior within an experimental class setting. In W. C. Becker (Ed.), *An empirical basis for change in education.* Chicago: Science Research Associates, 1971.

Watzlawik, P., Weakland, J., & Fisch, R. *Change: Principles of problem formation and problem resolution.* New York: Norton, 1974.

Winnet, R., & Winkler, R. Current behavior modification in the classroom: Be still, be quiet, be docile. *Journal of Applied Behavior Analysis,* 1972, *5,* 499-504.

Chapter 4

INDIVIDUAL-PROCESS CONSULTATION

Kenneth Heller, Ph.D.
John Monahan, Ph.D.

Consultation theorists typically distinguish between client-centered, consultee-centered, and program-centered consultation (Mannino & Shore, 1972). In other words, consultation can focus on an agency's clients, staff, or program. Client-centered case consultation, described in this book as the *educational model*, is most frequently practiced and is most familiar to specialists in all fields. Consultee-centered consultation, the focus of this chapter and also referred to as the *individual-process model*, has greater potential for changing attitudes and behavior but can raise ethical issues if not practiced with full awareness and consent of consultees. Program-centered or system consultation has the greatest potential for affecting community change. Unfortunately it is also the most difficult form of consultation, requiring the greatest understanding of community functioning.*

In individual-process consultation, the presenting problem may involve a particular case but the focus of consultation is on the consultee's difficulties with the case. The shift in focus may not be noticed by the consultee since the content of the discussion may remain centered about a case, but the consultant is using the medium of the case to improve a deficiency assumed to be present in the consultee. As described by Caplan (1970), the focus of consultation moves to the consultee when the problem is due to *a lack of knowledge or skill* (leading to an educational model) or to a temporary loss in self-confidence or a lapse in professional objectivity (leading to an individual-process model).

---

*The material for this chapter is adapted from K. Heller, and J. Monahan, *Psychology and Community Change,* Dorsey Press, Homewood, Ill., 1977, pp. 208-221 and 260-263, by permission of the authors.

When a problem is due to a lack of knowledge or skill, consultants often vary as to how they deal with these deficiencies. Some offer direct training in the problem areas; others refrain from direct intervention, believing that deficiencies in knowledge and skill are more appropriately dealt with through the normal channels of agency supervision. This chapter will not deal with work problems associated with lack of knowledge or skill. Instead the focus will be on issues associated with the consultant's approach to personal feelings of consultees that may interfere with their work—what Caplan called "lapses in professional objectivity."

Work problems due to lapses in professional objectivity can be difficult to handle. If the consultee is aware of personal involvement with the case, this topic can be approached directly in consultation. Personal feelings of anger, frustration, or disappointment can be discussed and viewed as natural responses to difficult work circumstances. A frequently occurring myth in human service organizations is that "true professionals" must not allow themselves to develop personal feelings toward their clients. Thus when natural feelings of frustration and anger arise, there is no organizational vehicle established to help work through these feelings. They are suppressed to avoid the label of being "foolish," "soft," or "unprofessional." The consultant can perform an important service by helping consultees accept and constructively use personal feelings that develop in the normal course of their work. If these feelings can be dealt with in a group setting, so much the better, for the consultees then can build their own support group that can function independently after the consultant terminates his or her services.

Knoblock and Goldstein (1971) discussed workshops with teachers in which the participants were encouraged to talk about the personal satisfactions and frustrations in their particular work settings. The authors described one such group as follows:

> Our teachers wanted to communicate that they could represent themselves as complex individuals. To be sure, they also felt they had good ideas about what could happen in schools with children and teachers. Even more importantly, they believed they had many skills and talents other than teaching skills. Many are talented and creative people who outside of the school pursue many avocations but within the school are asked to turn those off and run the ship as usual.
>
> In a summer workshop dealing with interpersonal competence, a group of teachers began to discuss poetry. One of the participants began to bring her poems to class, some of them inspired by the workshop and its participants. Two things were startling about this experience. One was the very fact that such creative people and behavior were neither acknowledged nor provided for in their school jobs. The other was that their degree of animation over such "avocational interests" was far more intense and involving than their teaching activities in the classroom.

It would seem from what our group and other teachers report that it is not sufficient to develop a personal and professional life which focuses exclusively on children. Teachers are equally concerned with responding to other adults and in turn being responded to by their colleagues.

In short, teachers would like very much to function as resources within the schools. How paradoxical it is that so many teachers do not see themselves as resources within their own classrooms, but rather as keepers of the peace, curriculum and school tradition. (Knoblock & Goldstein, 1971, pp. 13-14).

The function of the workshops in the Knoblock and Goldstein example was to provide a vehicle for teachers to share their feelings about their personal involvement in their work as one way of combatting professional loneliness. As long as no one is talking about job frustrations, it is very easy to assume erroneously that "everyone is satisfied, so I must be the oddball." The realization that dissatisfaction is shared can be a spark for corrective action to improve the work climate. Even if improvement is not likely, recognizing that satisfaction may have to come from avocational interests is still a valuable lesson that will probably improve overall life satisfaction.

How Open Should the Consultant Be In Confronting Consultee Feelings and Conflicts?

When consultees are unaware of personal involvement in their work, the dilemma for the consultant is whether to bring these feelings into conscious awareness or to deal with them more indirectly by discussing the relevant conflict-arousing issues through the medium of the case, that is, by focusing on the behavior of the consultee's client. This indirect approach is recommended by Caplan, who developed techniques of dealing with personal conflicts in consultees through displacement (see Caplan, 1970, pp. 125-222). As Caplan saw it, in his method the personality defenses of the consultee are not disturbed since he or she is never required to confront or examine personal feelings or the reasons for overinvolvement with the case. Only the client's personality and reactions are discussed. The problem may be the consultee's, but it is discussed as if it were the client's problem exclusively.

Caplan described the displacement technique in his description of consultation with an elementary school teacher (Caplan, 1970, pp. 140-142). The girl in question (Jean) had become a disciplinary problem, although her behavior had been trouble-free during the first half of the semester. Description of the onset of the problem by the teacher revealed that the change had occurred about the time of the first parent conference, when the teacher had discovered that Jean was the younger sister of a girl she had taught 3 years earlier. After the vacation following the parent conference, Jean's behavior began to deteriorate rapidly. The consultant remembered that this teacher consulted him earlier in the year about another girl in the class who was said to be suffering from a learning disorder and who also was described as someone's younger sister.

> The consultant did not know anything about the teacher's personal life, but he hazarded a guess to himself that she probably had a younger sister with whom she had been involved in unresolved conflicts similar in pattern to those she was now imposing on the case of Jean. In this regard, it appeared particularly significant that Jean became a problem to the teacher only after she discovered that she was "a younger sister." It also seemed that Jean's poor behavior occurred only in class with that teacher and was apparently a reaction to the teacher's method of handling her. (Caplan, 1970, p. 141)

The consultant did not begin a discussion of the teacher's personal life to find the suspected unresolved conflict. Instead he discussed the problem as if it were Jean's: that Jean was worried about being a younger sister and was afraid that the teacher would constantly compare her with her successful older sister.

> He pointed out that her behavior had regressed following the teacher's interview with her mother before Christmas, during which they had discussed her older sister. He put forward the hypothesis that after this interview the mother had told Jean that the teacher had been very fond of the older sister and remembered her quite vividly, and had possibly told her that the teacher hoped Jean would be as successful a student. The consultant then involved the teacher in a discussion of what this might have meant to Jean, and the nature of the conflict that might have been set up in her mind, so that she now might imagine that the teacher was continually comparing her with her older sister. The teacher, in this discussion, began to identify with the consultant, reversing roles and empathically imagining how Jean felt as a younger sister. . . . The consultant then posed the management problem as being for the teacher to work out ways of convincing Jean that her teacher was not a representative of her family constellation, and that Jean was a person in her own right and not just a "younger sister."
>   During the consultation session, the teacher quite suddenly made a switch in her patterned perceptions of Jean and began to talk about her as a child struggling to overcome in the classroom her misperceptions of her teacher. She then began to plan various alternative ways of dealing with her. . . .
>   During the remainder of the school year this teacher asked for consultation about two other cases neither one of which was a "younger sister." She gave follow-up reports on Jean, whose behavior

disorder had apparently completely resolved within three to four weeks following the second consultation discussion about her problems. (Caplan, 1970, p. 142)

Caplan's displacement approach has the advantage of reducing defensiveness in that the consultees may become suspicious and anxious and may avoid future contacts if the consultant approaches emotional issues directly. The fear that mental health professionals are ''out to psychoanalyze you'' becomes confirmed if consultees are led into emotional confrontation without warning. Even forewarned, potential consultees may see discussions that move into personal reactions as a violation of the consultation contract. Direct discussion of personal involvement, however, can be supported by the argument that bringing feelings into awareness can be an aid to learning and that learning without awareness is not very effective. In this sense, indirect methods may be too subtle. The main point of the consultant's message may never be received if it is made by analogy, conveyed in a parable, or presented by other similar indirect means.

The problem can be summarized as follows. Dealing with the personal involvement of the consultee in a work problem by helping to encourage its conscious recognition should lead to a more effective resolution as the consultee learns to accept and deal with the emotions engendered by the work situation. Not all consultees, however, are ready for emotional learning experiences, and some may become anxious or attempt to flee consultation if it becomes apparent that this is the consultant's goal. Indirect methods of consultation that deal with personal involvement but never bring it to awareness would seem better suited to these instances. Here, too, there are drawbacks. The effectiveness of learning without awareness can be questioned. An ethical question can be raised concerning indirect methods in that consultants are forced to work under false pretenses. The focus is on change in the consultees, but the consultants must take great pains to keep this intent secret and must steadfastly maintain that they are talking only about the consultees' case.

There is no completely satisfactory resolution to the difficulties raised here. It is our own personal belief that direct methods of consultation for consultee-centered problems are to be preferred when they can be utilized. In organizations marked by a lack of openness and a high degree of defensiveness among line staff, the consultant must seriously consider the options available. One possibility is to deal with problems involving a lapse in professional objectivity only with those who are open to change and are willing to examine their own contributions to their work problems. It could be argued that consultation should be offered only when receptivity is high.

The problem is that it is difficult to ignore lapses in professional objectivity if they occur in more defensive care givers who occupy important positions in the socialization and care-giving network of a community. One could not expect to have a major impact on the lives of children if their teachers were ignored as being too resistant to change. It is in these special instances when the need for intervention is particularly acute that we believe indirect methods of consultee-centered consultation have some value.

A Special Case of Consultee-Centered Consultation: Theme-Interference Reduction

We have already seen that Caplan advocated dealing with personal problems of consultees through displacement of the problem onto case material. As a psychoanalyst, Caplan believed that such indirection is even more important for personal problems associated with "repressed impulses." For such "unconscious" problems that represent an interfering theme in the client's work, Caplan devised a special technique that he labeled *theme-interference reduction*. The technique will be described at this point because of its prominence and because, as we shall explain shortly, we believe it has some value in dealing with untested stereotypes that can affect worker performance.

Caplan posited that a lack of professional objectivity in an otherwise competent consultee can be caused by the sudden emergence of a heretofore successfully repressed impulse. The original repression occurred because, in his or her own psychological development, the consultee was led to expect severe punishment if the impulse in question was expressed. Now, years later, the consultee comes across a case with a similar theme. The case disturbs the defensive equilibrium that the consultee has established, raises considerable tension in the consultee, and leads to the lapse in professional objectivity. The consultee is upset because only an unfortunate consequence can be seen as the outcome to this particular case. The case is "doomed" because it represents the sense of doom the consultee anticipates personally, should unacceptable impulses emerge.

Caplan's technique is to demonstrate to the consultee that the case that represents the prohibited theme can possibly escape the doomed outcome. By indirection, the message to the consultee is that those with similar problems (including the consultee) need not be doomed. This message cannot be stated directly, however. Doing so would be to confront the consultee with the repressed, prohibited theme, an upsetting personal experience that in addition would probably be ineffective. Confronted with unconscious material, the consultee would most likely not recognize the theme, deny its personal relevance, become anxious and then angry at the consultant.

Helping the consultee become aware of the interfering theme more gradually is also not recommended. This more gradual procedure would not be traumatic to the consultee, but it would bring the consultation relationship closer to psychotherapy—which is rarely sanctioned in consultation and would represent an inefficient use of time. Except for the displaced problem, the consultee is assumed to be functioning adequately. Becoming involved in psychotherapy would further restrict the range of other problems to which the consultant could be exposed. There is simply no time to develop a long-term therapeutic relationship with one consultee, nor is it appropriate in consultation.

The technique of theme-interference reduction is designed to reduce the psychological interference produced by the problem case without the consultee's becoming aware that the difficulty in the case is a result of his or her own unresolved conflict. The consultant keeps the discussion constantly on the case and in this sense deals with the unconscious conflicts of the consultee by displacing them onto the case. The technique involves finding the interfering theme or themes in the case material by monitoring the consultee's interview behavior for signs of increasing anxiety, overinvolvement, confusion, or any other unusual professional conduct. The anxiety-arousing material is never dealt with directly. Once it is discovered, the consultant moves away from the "hot" topic only to return to it later to discover the full extent of the theme. In Caplanian language, the consultant is attempting to "identify a syllogistic theme with its definable Initial Category and Inevitable Outcome" (Caplan, 1970, p. 154) so as to break the link between the two.

The *initial category* refers to the stereotyped view of the case that the consultee maintains because it reflects his or her own unacceptable impulses; hence the consultee cannot think about the case clearly without anxiety. The *inevitable outcome* refers to the sense of foreboding about the cases's outcome the consultee feels because it relates to the unrecognized belief that all persons with similar unacceptable impulses (including himself or herself) are "doomed."

According to Caplan, theme interference can be reduced in two ways. The first approach, called *unlinking*, attempts to change the consultee's perception of the client so as to remove the client from the initial category—in other words, unlinking the client from the consultee's theme. If the initial category was "all people who masturbate excessively," unlinking would involve convincing the consultee that the level of masturbation exhibited by the client was not excessive for a boy of his age. Unlinking is considered a cardinal error in consultation technique, for even though the consultee may gain temporary relief from anxiety, the unconscious theme is left intact at full strength.

A more lasting benefit is claimed for the second consultation approach. The consultant agrees with the categorization of the client as fitting the initial category, but then proceeds to reexamine the evidence for the inevitable outcome. If the consultant can open the consultee's perception to the recognition that other more beneficial outcomes are not only possible but perhaps more likely, again consultee tension lessens but this time because the effects of the interfering theme are being reduced. In Caplain's words, "Because the theme applies also to him, the invalidation of the syllogism for his client also has an effect of significantly reducing the consultee's tension regarding his own underlying conflict" (Caplan, 1970, p. 149).

REINTERPRETING THEME-INTERFERENCE REDUCTION AS A PROCEDURE FOR DEALING WITH STEREOTYPED ATTITUDES

Several questions can be put to this approach. First, do unconscious conflicts exist, and if so are they capable of interfering with the work capacity of a consultee in so circumscribed a manner? Remember that the assumption is that the psychological adjustment of the consultee is adequate; the effects of unconscious conflict are seen only by its displacement on the case. If the conflict is strong, why does it not show in other behaviors of the consultee? If it is weak, why does it produce so pronounced an effect with this *one* case, and why do the otherwise intact defenses of the consultee not help in providing a successful resolution without the necessity of consultation intervention?

A second line of questions concern the avoidance of consultee awareness. Not only is the consultee unaware that personal conflicts are the subject of consultation, but the consultant also does not know the full, detailed content of these conflicts and is prohibited by the technique from finding out. The consultant knows their content only in a general way by noting the topics that produce the most consultee tension and anxiety. Consultation moves along without either party knowing the content of the conflicts to which it is addressed. That it is moving on the right track can be determined only from the drop in tension level exhibited by the consultee. Considering the wide array of factors that can reduce tension in the consultee (e.g., increased rapport with and trust of the consultant, unlinking, a new cognitive grasp of the case having nothing to do with unconscious conflict), it is difficult to see how the presence of an unconscious conflict can ever be truly determined. Avoidance of consultee awareness raises other issues: Is it ethical to work on another's conflicts without explicit permission? And, once it becomes generally known that consultants are looking for unconscious conflicts in consultees, this latter group, becoming aware of the consultants' intent, are no longer proper subjects for theme-interference reduction. Finally, the coordinate relationship of two professionals, consultant and consultee, working on a common problem together is destroyed when one of them is all the while secretly tampering with the psyche of the other.

If it is removed from its psychoanalytic underpinning, there may be some useful implications to Caplan's technique. Consider the possibility that a consultee may at times be suffering from a stereotype. The stereotype might be a reflection of cultural attitudes learned in early socialization, such as that blacks are sexually promiscuous, men who don't work are lazy, masturbation leads to insanity, women who have extramarital affairs can't be good mothers. Or the stereotyped attitude could result from an unfortunate personal experience that has been blown up out of proportion and is now the source of an inappropriately overgeneralized negative attitude.

Regardless of their origins, stereotyped views are rarely accessible to change through direct attack or challenge. We agree with Caplan that excluding one individual from a stereotype can change an attitude toward that individual, but the stereotype still may be left intact. The process Caplan called *unlinking* involves removing a case from the consultee's general stereotype, and we feel that it is less preferred as a method of influencing stereotyped attitudes. A much better possibility would be to expand the consultee's perceptual field by broadening the view of members of the stereotyped group. This can be done by demonstrating that one member of the stereotyped group whom the consultee knows well (the case) has unrecognized assets. This is essentially what Caplan's method does when it demonstrates that an unfortunate or "doomed" outcome is not inevitable.

In summary, we feel that Caplan's procedures are enmeshed in a psychoanalytic rationale that hides their more general utility. We doubt that many consultees are bothered by unconscious conflicts that operate in the circumscribed way that Caplan's method requires. This does not invalidate the technique, only the theory. Caplan's procedure is one way of dealing with overgeneralized and untested stereotyped attitudes. In the name of reducing interfering themes, Caplan and his coworkers may be obtaining a consultee's effective relief and movement on a case because the consultee is no longer trapped by a perception of restricted alternatives available to the client. Expanding these alternatives can serve to broaden one's picture of the entire situation. This is essentially what Levy referred to as psychological interpretation, "a redefining or restructuring of the situation through the presentation of an alternative description of some behavior datum" (Levy, 1963, p. 5). Theme interference reduction seems to be just such a process.

Thus far we have been focusing on understanding how to deal with personal feelings of consultees. At this point, we would like to summarize our views of the general process of consultation by highlighting what we see as basic assumptions that are shared by the various consultation perspectives.

SUMMARY OF CONSULTATION ASSUMPTIONS

From our point of view, regardless of specialized content or techniques, the essential similarity among consultants of the various perspectives is that they are all oriented toward a similar goal, that is, to affect positive changes in essential human service and socialization institutions through program modification and by increasing the psychological sophistication and work capacity of the primary care givers within these institutions. As applied to human service organizations the following assumptions can be derived from the various consultation perspectives:

1. Very few problems in real life are exclusively psychological in nature. The most troubling problems are those with complex determinants, of which the psychological component, while significant, is just one among many. There is little gained when clients with difficulties in living are "taken over" by personnel in the mental health sphere. If anything, there are distinct disadvantages to labeling problems exclusively in mental health terms, not only because of the adverse consequences for the individual so labeled or because the mental health professions could never develop the work force needed to deal with all those who would then be thrust upon them. An even more critical disadvantage is that mental health professions do not control the tangible real-life reinforcements necessary for changing individual or corporate behavior in our society. By themselves they do not possess the leverage to affect social contingencies impinging upon individuals.

2. Communities have well-developed systems for providing human services. The greatest benefit can be obtained if mental health personnel use their expertise to ensure that these services are administered in such a way that they do not contribute to conditions that would increase the likelihood of producing mental health casualties. It is assumed that since primary care givers and agents of social control constantly deal with problems of behavior, the more they know about psychological development and the principles of behavior, the more likely will it be that they will take psychologically sound, humane action.

3. Considering the great array of human service professions, consultants will realize the greatest preventive potential in their work if they affiliate with units in the community that have primary responsibility for

psychological and social development and that deal with young populations still in their formative years. There would be greater preventive potential in working with administrative officials who determine policy and programs with regard to school behavior or with teachers making mental health referrals than with clinics to whom such referrals are made. There would be similar advantages in working with probation or police departments rather than in correctional facilities for convicted offenders, or on an intake unit that screens disordered individuals brought to a hospital as compared with hospital wards for chronic mental patients.

4. The consultant's long-term goal is to obtain some permanent change in the consultee or the consultee's institution. There would be little economic gain if all cases with a psychological component were called to a consultant's attention. Neither would there be any particular advantage if consultants were sought out only for some particular difficulties, and over time the nature of the problems called to their attention remained the same. Consultants hope that their efforts will go beyond the specific case material brought to their attention. It is in this sense that consultation can be thought of as a radiating process (Kelly, 1970). Improved functioning by consultees or better programs developed by consultee institutions affect the client populations who are beneficiaries of the improved service. Thus the impact of consultation is most appropriately measured, not just by changes in consultees, but also by changes in those significant others who are served by the consultees.

5. A consultant must have a background in some substantive content area that relates to understanding the human condition. It should be clear that consultation does not denote a new profession independent of others. The area of specialization need not be the traditional mental health professions—some would argue that the mental health fields represent too narrow a view of community life. Whatever the area, it must have a body of knowledge and skill that the consultant can use in orienting the direction of work. Nothing is sadder to see in the field than a consultant who has nothing to offer the host organization and who seems to assume that his or her mere presence alone will "make things happen."

The substantive areas from which mental health consultants might draw are quite varied, including the range from urban planning, sociology, and public health nursing to the more traditional mental health "team": psychiatry, psychology, and psychiatric social work. Caplan (1970) suggested that the consultant's particular expertise is in the mental health area. There are, however, consultants who would prefer to describe their work as "psychological" or as "behavioral" rather than accept the language of health and illness. Other consultants would point out that their expertise is in "problem solving," so that the help they provide is not circumscribed by a particular type of problem. Instead they teach problem-solving skills that should be applicable to work difficulties of almost any content.

6. *Not all human service workers can benefit from consultation.* Several problems confront those attempting to develop a program of intervention based upon the preceding assumptions that are not typically addressed by consultation theorists. To begin with, one may ask whether it is reasonable to expect non-mental health personnel to perform psychological functions. The consultant *does* ask human service workers to concern themselves with the psychological components of their work. To those who respond that their training does not equip them to dabble in the psyche of others, the consultant replies that their normal work functions are made more difficult when attempts are not made to understand and deal with behavior patterns of clients. There is accumulating evidence to support the consultant's claim that non-mental health personnel can be trained to respond in psychologically helpful ways (Guerney, 1969).

However, not all can be so trained. Some individuals who have gravitated to community care-giving and socialization roles still may be so deficient in interpersonal sensitivity and skill that no amount of training will improve their functioning. These individuals would probably do less harm if they did not attempt to intervene in a psychologically meaningful manner. We are not referring to consultees who simply differ in values or interpersonal style from their consultants. Most consultants already know that they must guard against the tendency to assume that all who disagree with their mission are of dubious mental health. We are referring to those individuals whose entry into a human service field was clearly in error and who are unamenable to change by a consultant despite his or her best effort.

All human service professions (including the mental health professions) contain a small minority of members whose adjustment is tenuous and who should not be in work that requires sensitivity and responsiveness to others. Undoubtedly the professions themselves could do better screening those who apply to their training program. The mental health consultant who finds these individuals in working with agencies, has very few options. The point we are making here is simply that consultation should not be expected to be effective under all circumstances. There are primary care givers who are not amenable to change. In working for institutional change from within organizational structures, the consultant hopes and expects that the majority will be basically competent and psychologically healthy and will be responsive to improving their work performance.

REFERENCES

Caplan, G. *The theory and practice of mental health consultation.* New York: Basic Books, 1970.

Guerney, B. G., Jr. (Ed.). *Psychotherapeutic agents: New roles for nonprofessionals, parents and teachers.* New York: Holt, Rinehart & Winston, 1969.

Kelly, J. G. The quest for valid preventive interventions. In C. D. Spielberger (Ed.), *Current topics in clinical and community psychology* (Vol. 2). New York: Academic Press, 1970, pp. 183-207.

Knoblock, P., & Goldstein, A. P. *The lonely teacher.* Boston: Allyn and Bacon, 1971.

Levy, L. H. *Psychological interpretation.* New York: Holt, Rinehart & Winston, 1963.

Mannino, R. V., & Shore, M. F. Research in mental health consultation. In S. E. Golann & C. Eisdorfer (Eds.), *Handbook of community mental health.* New York: Appleton-Century-Crofts, 1972, pp. 755-777.

Chapter 5

SYSTEM-PROCESS
MENTAL HEALTH MODELS

Richard A. Schmuck, Ph.D.

Social systems shape what people's wants are, how they view themselves, and how they actually behave toward one another. Along with this assumption about human behavior, the chapter is guided by two others: that many mental health difficulties arise because of people's participation in unhealthy social systems and that acting on social system health itself as a change target offers a promising, indirect strategy for ameliorating individual mental illness.

The health of any living system depends on how effectively it carries out optimal transactions with its changing environment as well as on how effectively it maintains relationships among its internal parts. In relation to the latter, living systems are made up of subsystems that process inputs, throughputs, and outputs of different forms of matter, energy, and information. Discerning the health of subsystem processes and intervening to upgrade them, particularly in relation to the quality of human life within social systems, offers both an intellectual and a tactical challenge to the mental health consultant.

CHARACTERISTICS OF SOCIAL SYSTEMS

According to Miller (1978), there are seven levels of living systems, ranging in scope from cells and organs; through individuals, groups, and organizations; to nation-states and supranational systems. At any level a system is a bounded array of interdependent subsystems and components, devoted to the achievement of some goal or goals, with the components maintained in equilibrium in relation to one another and to the environment by means of both regular internal procedures and feedback from the environment about the impact of system action. This chapter is particularly concerned with groups and organizations, and we should at the outset distinguish between variables characteristic of individuals (the usual focus of mental health) and those that typify social systems (groups and organizations). We shall see, for example, that providing interventions with an individual in psychotherapy by assuming that pathology resides within that person is very different from trying to help the same individual to function effectively within a social system. The latter intervention will require taking into account system norms, structures, and procedures.

Norms, Structures, and Procedures

In attempting to understand human nature, psychologists typically have focused on perceptions, cognitions, affect, motives, and actions of individuals, and various types of psychotherapy have given different weight to these several aspects. In contrast, the targets of social system interventions to enhance organizational health are at a qualitatively different level of human nature, requiring the analytic tools of the social psychologist. Groups and organizations are constituted of norms, structures, and procedures that are merely analogous to, but not the same as, the individual's affects, cognitions, and behaviors.

Norms cannot be measured, as the psychologist might, by summing the attitudes of the participants in a social system as if one were polling each individual separately and adding the responses. Since norms are *shared* expectations about how a system member ought to think, feel, and behave in relation to a particular issue, the dynamics of sharedness must be assessed. Doing so requires noting that two or more persons believe that the others hold expectations similar to theirs and that all expect one another to behave according to the content of those expectations.

Thus norms are constituted of implicit or explicit interpersonal exchanges between two or more system participants, with neophytes being socialized into the norms through listening, observing, modeling, venturing, and receiving feedback. There might be a norm within a welfare department that no one should comment on differences in the competencies of staff nor behave as though differences in job performance existed. Each staff member might privately hold very different attitudes on this issue, causing the naive consultant trouble if only the private views are assessed. An attempt by the consultant to intervene with a group discussion about job performance would very likely create more tension than it would resolve. And new staff members might place themselves in jeopardy unless they quickly picked up on the pressures to avoid both comparisons of members' performances and detailed discussions about effectiveness of the agency.

Structures also represent more than a mere summing of the individual's cognitive maps about the organization. Structures involve visible networks of interdependencies, sequences of interaction, and behavioral exchanges that constitute a larger social reality than any individual participant can perceive. Structures may be more easily and directly assessed than norms because the latter so frequently are implicit or preconscious. System structures are typically physical and vivid; they can be assessed through observations of person-to-person interactions, group formations, routings of memos and correspondence, paths of telephone calls, and the like. In a public school, the consultant might discover that a secretary or an administrative assistant acts as the informal center of communication, with most messages to the principal, custodian, or central office going through him or her. Assessing system structures often becomes difficult, both because of the complex logistics required in monitoring the massive structures of bureaucracies and because of the not-so-obvious informal structures involving influence, friendship, and social support.

Procedures, the third basic characteristic of social systems, are formal activities based on tradition or law for accomplishing the tasks and the maintenance of an organization. Meetings are called in a particular way and run according to some agreed-upon patterns, records are kept in standard forms, new members go through standard routines, job evaluations are executed in certain fashions, etc. Procedures also are guided by both formal and informal norms. Thus, for example, there may be high agreement in a police department about how a drunk should be handled, even if rules about such a circumstance may not be written.

Generic Subsystems

The norms, structures, and procedures of an organization can further be characterized by subsystems common to all organizations. Katz and Kahn (1978) defined these as generic and viewed them as being concerned with production, support, maintenance, adaptation, and management.

Production subsystems are concerned with the work of the organization. They constitute the throughput processes of transforming either energy and matter (such as metals into machinery in an industrial organization) or information (such as knowledge for clients in service-oriented organizations). Supportive subsystems are closely related to production, carrying out transactions both to procure appropriate resources (raw materials or information) for production and to dispose of the output. Maintenance subsystems exist alongside, keeping production flowing efficiently and effectively by attending to human motivation, accuracy, and committed effort (such as in the work of personnel or staff development departments). They build the interdependence needed to facilitate continuous task accomplishment through recruitment, socialization, training, rewards, sanctions, and the like.

The production, support, and maintenance subsystems are concerned with getting the work done well. They represent the organization as it is functioning now rather than what it might become. Since they turn inward to the throughput, they are not attuned to demands of a rapidly changing environment. Adaptive subsystems, conversely, are required to look outward, devoting energies to anticipating environmental alterations and coping with them by carrying out such activities as long-range planning, market research, and product development. The research and evaluation section of a school district often performs the functions of the adaptive subsystem.

For the production, support, maintenance, and adaptive functions to work in an integrated fashion, coordination is required. Managerial subsystems involving the administrators of a system offer coordination along with the control and direction needed to keep the organization on course. Some of the managerial functions are guided by regulatory mechanisms involving uses of information about outputs and feedback about the impact of the outputs, such as when the administrators of a central office in a school district feed data about student achievement back to school staffs. Management also includes authority structures for problem solving and decision making through which policies, rules, and regulations are determined and monitored. The notorious staff meeting in virtually any organization is a case in point.

Formal and Informal Aspects

The generic subsystems must be articulated to accomplish the organization's primary tasks and to satisfy human needs sufficiently to keep the organization on course. Thus in a hospital, well-trained nurses must be given appropriate medicines and clear diagnostic information about particular patients in a manner that is both systematic and sensitive to the professional norms of nursing. To put it in theoretical terms, the norms, structures, and procedures of the subsystems of the hospital must be so constituted that they ensure the predictability, efficiency, and coordination of the efforts of the technicians, doctors, nurses, and patients. In even the most efficient hospital, those formal aspects of the organization can only partly satisfy the work-related motivations and interests of all the nurses, technicians, and doctors. Even the socialization functions executed within maintenance subsystems of personnel and staff development only partly satisfy the motives of organizational members, because those functions are shaped primarily in light of the hospital's formal tasks involving patient care and only secondarily by personal needs.

In virtually every formal organization, including welfare departments, public schools, the police, and hospitals, there inevitably arises a conflict between the task focus of the organization and the psychological desires of the members. These divergent pulls in social systems reflect the rational and the emotional side of human nature. Rationality is characterized by the norms, structures, and procedures of the generic subsystems, but the emotional aspects of human behavior frequently are de-emphasized, even suppressed, by the organization's task focus. The pressures for producing a lot, getting tasks done on time in a certain order, and doing particular tasks according to narrowly defined standards can frustrate members' needs for influence, autonomy, and creativity. Or, altering people's jobs to enhance production and to cut costs frequently disrupts meeting friends at coffee breaks, participating in car pools, and the like. As a consequence, informal structures, which offer legitimate avenues for emotional expression, develop and exist alongside and with the formal subsystems. Cliques meeting during coffee breaks or breaking together for lunch are common-place. These informal structures take on norms and procedures of their own that frequently can be in opposition to the smooth functioning of the formal subsystems.

The multiple aspects of a social system are illustrated by the alternative school described in Figure 5-1.

HEALTHY SYSTEM PROCESSES

In this chapter the concept of health is not employed to represent an absence of illness or disease. Rather the concept of health is used, in the spirit of preventive medicine, to depict positive well-being, optimal functioning, and a state of ideal human affairs toward which to strive. With this in mind, system health can be analyzed at three levels: organizational problem solving, subsystem effectiveness, and the individual as a self-actualizing participant.

Organizational Problem Solving

A healthy organization does not merely survive in its environment; it goes beyond to cope adequately over the long haul and to develop and extend its coping abilities. In particular, a healthy organization is continuously solving problems that arise either because factions from the outside are pressing for change or because new goals are being established within

	NORMS		STRUCTURES		PROCEDURES	
	Formal	Informal	Formal	Informal	Formal	Informal
PRODUCTION	Individualized instruction will be offered whenever feasible	Teachers do not share their teaching techniques with one another	No class is bigger than 25 or smaller than 10	The English and Social Studies teachers drink together on Friday afternoons	Achievement tests are taken every April by the 9th and 11th graders	Some teachers keep grade books and make lesson plans even though they are not required
SUPPORT	To enroll, a prospective student must meet certain criteria	Parents of this school go to board meetings more than do parents from other schools	A committee of administrators, teachers, and parents visit elementary schools to talk about the school	Alumni met one year after graduation	A standard application form is filled out by prospective students and their parents	Parents that go to board meetings bring information about other schools to administrators and teachers
MAINTENANCE	New teachers meet with principal frequently during their first 6 weeks	Teachers discipline misbehaving students even when they are outside the classroom	The whole staff attends a retreat together three times a year to review their program	New staff members do not have close friends on the staff	All teachers serve as organizers and monitors at school assemblies football games, dances, etc.	The custodian walks around the school grounds twice a day
ADAPTIVE	Administrators and teachers share an interest in the fortunes of the school's graduates	Administrators and teachers do not plan together for the future	The principal meets regularly with a district-wide administrator committee for long-range planning	Head of Women's Physical Education is married to Assistant Superintendent in charge of Program Evaluation	Alumni receive questionnaires once a year on what they are doing	Alumni periodically make unplanned visits to the school
MANAGEMENT	The principal and department heads tell one another about school-wide problems they perceive	The principal and department heads do not give critical feedback to one another or to teachers	The school is organized in departments with an administrative cabinet over the departments	The principal and a few department heads belong to the same bowling team	All new teachers for the first 3 years are involved in an MBO program with the principal	The principal gets to school early and leaves late.

Figure 1
Examples from an Alternative School

the organization. Organizational problem solving means reaching for, remaining open to, and filtering information from both outside and inside the organization; examining information over a period of time; becoming aware of changes that occur; and attempting to predict changes to come. It also means employing systematic procedures to create solutions, changing a normal mode of operation to solve new or anticipated problems, and continuously rechecking to see whether movement toward goals improves. Such effective problem solving can be seen in the alternative school in which a staff-parent steering committee gathers information from both the parents and the staff at large, carefully analyzes that information, and eventually takes action upon it.

A healthy organization makes use of a host of resources, both external and internal, to aid in solving problems and in being responsive to new demands. Buckley (1967) referred to an organization's repertoire of usable or potential resources as its *variety pool*, a concept that includes not only individual skills, information, and interests, but also the organizational norms, structures, and procedures that may exist. Although many organizations possess a rich variety of resources, the healthy organization makes use of most that it has and establishes ways of continuously uncovering new ones.

Subsystem Effectiveness

For organizations to engage effectively in adaptive problem solving with their environment, they must have subsystems that are effectively functioning in themselves. Subsystem effectiveness may be determined in two ways: first, by exploring the nature of a subsystem's norms, structures, and procedures, and second, by diagnosing the sorts of articulation, interdependence, and conflict management procedures connecting each subsystem with every other. Thus a hospital's system health increases to the extent that nurses on a ward are cooperative and helpful to one another, as well as to the degree that they quickly communicate to one another about modifications in the practices of the doctors and the technicians.

Effectively functioning subsystems have norms, structures, and procedures that integrate the formal and informal lives of the participants in the service of both goal achievement and social-emotional maintenance. Thus effectiveness of subsystems may be assessed by checking on their goal and role clarity, communicative accuracy and clarity, efficient agenda setting and meeting procedures, decision-making involvement and clarity, resource identification and use, cohesiveness and morale, and the presence of evaluation feedback loops across hierarchical levels. In particular, a diagnosis of effectiveness must be concerned with dovetailing of the formal and informal processes of the subsystem. When the informal processes, in the form of collegial relationships and norms, are not supportive of the formal missions, considerable interpersonal tension and discord can arise, hindering task performance of the participants. Worker sabotage in the form of reduced productivity and a lack of follow-through on tasks can be the result. Nurses who feel left out of a hospital's decision making may collude informally to drag their feet when it comes to complying with innovative practices, particularly if the nurses have developed friendly feelings toward one another and hostile feelings toward the demands of the doctors.

Healthy articulation across subsystems is of course a fundamental building block of organizational problem solving. When, for example, counselors and teachers at a secondary school do not see eye to eye on student discipline, considerable confusion and distress among the students can lead to an overload of problems for the administration, making it difficult for the administrators to deal effectively and efficiently with the central office and the parents. A diagnosis of effectivenes must be concerned with normative compatibility, structural interdependence, and procedural integration among the production, support, and maintenance subsystems; effective conflict management and resource sharing between these three subsystems and the adaptive subsystems; and optimal power sharing between the management subsystem and the other four subsystems. Moreover, at an interface between any of the subsystems, the consultant should search for role clarity, communicative accuracy, and the like.

Individuals as Self-Actualizing Participants

There are unquestionably links among satisfaction with organizational life, fulfillment of human motives, and the maintenance of self-esteem and self-respect. In attempting to understand these links, a substantial body of social-psychological research (e.g., Berlew, 1974; McClelland, 1958; Osgood & Suci, 1955) has led to the view that a central motive that involves striving for self-actualization also typically involves at least three motivational domains: (1) the striving for achievement, referred to as *competency, efficacy,* and *curiosity*; (2) the striving for power or influence in relation to others; and (3) the striving for affiliation, affection, and support. Typical emotions resulting from frustration of those motives are feelings of inferiority and incompetence; feelings of being put down, ignored, or losing control; and feelings of rejection, loneliness, and distrust.

Organizational participants will be more likely to remain motivated, have available more paths to further satisfaction, and be likely to become more productive if their achievement, power, and affiliation motives can be expressed and satisfied. Although collaborating and interacting with interdependent others in any of the generic subsystems can of course affect one's motive satisfaction and self-esteem, the consultant should look primarily to the production, supportive, and adaptive subsystems for achievement satisfactions; the maintenance subsystem for affiliation; and the management subsystem for power. Successful and satisfying role taking in any of the subsystems could enhance and buttress what Maslow referred to as *self-actualization* within the organization. Figure 5-2 summarizes the qualities of health with which to look at different loci within the system.

TARGETS FOR IMPROVING SYSTEM HEALTH

Confronting the challenge of improving system health commences by conceiving of organizations not as clusters of individuals working at separate tasks, but as interdependent subsystems made up of individual participants working together and moving into coordination with other sets of people from other subsystems as they move from task to task. The

Figure 2

SUMMARY OF HEALTHY SYSTEM PROCESSES

Locus Within the System	Qualities of Health
I N D I V I D U A L P R O C E S S E S	Achievement satisfaction, feelings of competency Power satisfactions, feelings of influence Affiliation satisfactions, feelings of affection Job satisfaction--self esteem
S U B S Y S T E M P R O C E S S E S	Goal and role clarity Communication accuracy and clarity Effective agenda setting and discussion Decision-making involvement and clarity Resource identification and use Cohesiveness and morale Evaluation and hierarchical feedback
R E L A T I O N S H I P S B E T W E E N S U B S Y S T E M S	Intergroup conflict management Optimal power sharing Functional interdependence Normative compatibility Structural integration

systemic nature of an organization lies in the coordinated interdependence (or lack of it) of subsystems of persons who work together in pursuit of organizational goals. The subsystems of adaptation, management, production, support, and maintenance typically are constituted of subgroups carrying forward a set of interdependent tasks. A starting point for system improvement requires understanding how the subsystems work, in their internal operations as well as their relationships with one another.

The Consultant's Stance

Although the organizational consultant takes the social system level as a conceptual starting point, many of the actual diagnostic measures will necessarily be constructed from questionnaires and interviews in which the perceptions, attitudes, and behavior of individuals are reported. Still it is important to note that the formal and informal norms, structures, and procedures residing in and between the subsystems guide the consultant's collection of individual data when making an assessment of system health. In studying the introduction of team teaching into an elementary school (an innovation in the production subsystem), a psychologically oriented consultant might concentrate on the teachers' personality needs for affiliation and autonomy, whereas a system-oriented consultant might focus on norms that legitimize collaborative planning, teaching, and evaluating. Just as the former could very well be concerned about compatibilities among the team members' values about education, the latter might be more concerned with goal and role clarity, communicative adequacy, and conflict management procedures within the team as well as between the team and other formal subgroups.

The contrasting diagnostic stances also relate to different strategies of consultation. The psychologically oriented consultant, for example, might be prone to employ a personnel-selection strategy, selecting the teachers of a team from those with higher needs for affiliation and with compatible educational values. Prospective team members who did not fit the pattern would be eliminated. In contrast, the system-oriented consultant would likely use an organization development strategy, placing emphasis on helping team members to use interpersonal skills in establishing group agreements about collaboration and a clear and appropriate role structure within the team. Individuals with different needs and values would be encouraged to find a place in the team's structure that would maximize their contribution to the unit's performance and maintenance.

Thus the system consultant assumes that, by making opportunities for system participants to learn interpersonal skills and to use them in relation to improving subsystem effectiveness, the organization can set in motion a change process through which collaboration and subgroup problem solving can establish the organization's capacity in solving its own problems. The following domains for improving system health undergird the stance taken by the system consultant to intervention. They represent the building blocks of system health.

Interpersonal Skills

The interpersonal skills of processing information, conceiving problems, and taking experimental action are the fundamental ingredients of effective subsystem functioning and organizational problem solving. Group problem solving requires gathering information, sharing and clarifying it, agreeing on the identification of a problem, conceiving and analyzing the problem, and having the ability to respond with experimental action.

Giving relevant information about one's role and tasks and eliciting task-related information from others constitute the two sides of processing information. They offer the paths by which subsystem members can create the common reality prerequisite to collaborative action. When emotions run high, however, as they frequently do as anxiety or disagreement surface, organization participants tend to close off channels of communication that ordinarily are open when things are going smoothly. In such circumstances, those who withhold information about their skills, ideas, and attitudes may deprive others of useful information and the subsystem of potential means of solving problems. Thus communication about relevant resources and constraints, particularly during high emotion, represents a basic interpersonal skill for improving system health.

Conceptualizing problems entails the search for available information about what is known of the present situation and the goals that are valued or preferred. In particular it requires specifying a discrepancy between current aspects of a situation and an ideal state and referring to that gap as the problem. Some common gaps occur when nurses prefer up-to-date information on patient progress and do not get it, or teachers prefer sustained task focus on the part of their students but instead experience considerable disruption and noise. Locating such gaps, acknowledging them, and accepting them as challenges require time, energy, creativity, and discipline. Above all, successful problem solving requires norms that support taking risks in uncovering heretofore unknown or ignored gaps. There is no certain way for all participants at all times to think of the steps, phases, and skills involved in conceiving problems, but the consultant should keep in mind that people tend to benefit from being conscious of the method they are using.

For a health system to flourish, accurate conceptions of problems, though necessary, are not sufficient. Organization participants must be capable of acting on their intentions and at the same time be aware of the impact of their actions on others. Many organization members can become more skilled at stating their role responsibilities, carrying them through, and being aware that they are doing so. Insofar as experimental responses and new role behaviors offer observable information that can be discussed and analyzed to conceive of still other problems, responding and acting are integrally and circularly connected to the skills of information exchange and problem processing.

Subsystem Norms and Roles

Subsystem processes can be conceived of as the complex interaction of norms and roles. *Norms* are shared expectations that a range of behavior within a specific context will either be approved, disapproved, or ignored. *Roles* are the set of norms specifying how a participant in a particular position should behave. Norms collected into a gestalt constitute the subsystem's culture, whereas an interrelated set of roles make up the subsystem's structure. Along with focusing on interpersonal skills, the system consultant looks toward making modifications in the subsystem's culture and structure to enhance system health.

The social-psychological character of norms is relevant to the consultant's scheme of intervention. First, they help to coordinate the subsystem's structure by causing behavior to be guided by common expectations, attitudes, and understandings. Second, norms can facilitate both the subsystem's viability and the individual's sense of well-being. Third, norms can promote a clear role structure by helping to specify the appropriate behaviors for each functionally separate task. Finally, for the individual participant, norms provide a basis for social reality, especially when objective reality is ambiguous, as it so often is for people working in the adaptive and the management subsystem.

Furthermore, although norms may act to resist system change, they can be gradually modified to bring about changes in tasks and roles. They can be altered when organization participants conjointly and simultaneously experiment with innovative ways of doing things and sustain these new actions long enough until all involved come to believe that their colleagues will accept and continue with the new patterns of role behavior. Such sustained, conjoint action is particularly important when the norms to be changed are associated with the interpersonal competencies or skills of individuals. Many interpersonal patterns and features of social structure can be modified if subsystem members explicitly make formal agreements conjointly (and this is always the point of departure for the system consultant), but patterns of interaction characterized by strong ego involvement may also require time-consuming one-to-one agreements supported by the consultant as a third party. The interpersonal agreements must subsequently be supported by other subsystem participants and legitimized through formation of new norms.

System Capacity for Problem Solving

Four clusters of interdependent, formal activities characterize a social system's capacity for problem solving. When functioning in a healthy fashion, these activities are legitimized and guided by appropriate norms, accomplished as a formal aspect of the structure, and acted out through regularly executed procedures. First is the systematic diagnosis of discrepancies between actual and ideal states that exist within the organization's environment, between its subsystems, within the subsystems, and between particular role takers. Second is proactive retrieval of appropriate resources from within and without the organization for the purpose of reducing the discrepancies specified during the diagnosis. Third is the rapid formation of ad hoc groups, frequently with members from several subsystems, that can efficiently and effectively use available resources to reduce the diagnosed discrepancies. Fourth is the self-analytic, formative evaluation of the preceding three clusters of activities.

A considerable degree of responsibility for organizing and executing systematic diagnoses falls to the adaptive and management subsystems. The former, which may, for example, be a marketing research unit, is the appropriate locus in the organization in which to search for diagnoses of the environment, whereas the latter, the line supervisors, for example, dwells more on diagnosing problems that might exist between subsystems. Each subsystem would typically be responsible for diagnosing its own internal discrepancies, but as a matter of fact the management subsystem typically shares this responsibility with each other subsystem. Proactive retrieval of resources represents a special responsibility of the supportive subsystem, particularly in relation to production, but here, too, the adaptive and management subsystems will play a part. The adaptive subsystem will be vigilant to resources that lie outside the system, whereas the management subsystem will facilitate resource exchange between and within the production, supportive, and maintenance subsystems. Facilitating formation of cross-subsystem, problem-solving subgroups also typically falls to the initiative of the management subsystem. At the same time, each subsystem will usually be expected to form its own internal subgroups for working on internal issues. Finally, the self-analytic evaluation of problem-solving processes would be executed to some degree within each subsystem, but again a considerable amount of the responsibility for organizing and facilitating system evaluation falls to the management subsystem.

System-process consultation aims to upgrade interpersonal skills, to clarify and refurbish subsystem norms and roles, and to develop an effective organizational capacity for solving problems on a continuous basis. It further aims to upgrade the quality of life in an organization in terms of facilitating development of norms, structures, and procedures within the subsystems that will help individual participants satisfy their achievement, power, and affiliation strivings. By so doing, the consultants strive to serve both the organization, in its productivity and maintenance, and the individual participants, in their self-actualization.

Offered here are some considerations about how the system-process consultant might proceed when intervening. Described here are some issues at the start-up of the consultation along with several alternative intervention designs.

Introduction and Contract Building

Consultants should be aware that what takes place during the introduction and contract-building phase foreshadows much of what is to come. If the system improvement effort is to be built on a solid base of participant support, it is crucial to gain at least a publicly delivered oral commitment from key members of all subsystems that will be participating in it. To this end, the critical importance of establishing relaxed rapport, credibility, trust, and legitimacy at the outset and of arriving at clear statements about goals, competencies, and shared expectations cannot be overemphasized. System-process consultants must be explicit about their role, the targets of system health (as spelled out earlier in this chapter), the project's budget, and the time they are expecting to devote to the project. The last is of supreme importance since system change requires time, often 2 or 3 years in many organizations. During start-up the consultant should also note the extent to which clients adopt a collaborative stance, as well as the extent to which they appear ready to collaborate with one another in new ways, since the length of time a system change effort will require will be strongly influenced by the amount of readiness for change in the client group.

Although a system-process consultant may initially be contacted by a role taker of any subsystem, introductory discussions should very soon occur between the consultant and key figures in the management subsystem. We have already noted in previous sections of this chapter the crucial roles played by members of the management subsystem in relation to organizational problem solving. At the same time, gaining approval and collaboration of the managers alone will not necessarily win commitment from others in the system. Indeed, the implication of collusion between the consultant and the managers could lead to the project's rapid demise. Consultants must keep in mind that they are working for system change through the subsystems and that introductory, contract-building sessions should be carried out with key members of each subsystem. The sessions may initially be arranged through key members of the management subsystem, but subsequent contacts often should be made independent of management participation. It will frequently be the case, in fact, that relationships between management and the other subsystems become the focus of considerable problem solving and innovation as the consultation moves along.

Although discussions of system characteristics, healthy system processes, the targets of system improvement, consultative designs, and intervention techniques characterize the initial phases, sound consultant-client relationships are not forged by agreement about intervention tasks alone. The consultant should remain aware that the dynamics of start-up and contract building often arouse intense feelings of suspicion and distrust, defensiveness and dissatisfaction, investment and caution, and vulnerability and reserve. Even though system change is the target, individual participants themselves will of course undergo the change process with their own thoughts and feelings. Directly acknowledging their thoughts and feelings about change as well as discussing them in direct, empathic ways can be a prime requisite for valid contract building and for a successful design.

Alternative Intervention Designs

The system-process consultant has a repertoire of macrodesigns and their microaspects. A macrodesign comprises the overall structure and outline, sequence of parts, and general forms through which activities flow. An example implied by the discussion earlier in this chapter would include upgrading interpersonal skills through training, changing subsystem norms through improving collaborative goal setting, and improving the organization's capacity for problem-solving through cross-subsystem confrontation and group agreements. Microaspects of a design refer to the specific activities played out during any limited period of consultation. These may include specific skill-development activities, group exercises, and innovative organizational procedures. Perhaps the most important of all microaspects is a systematic problem-solving sequence since it would fit into virtually all macrodesigns.

Several types of macrodesigns for system-process intervention—training, data feedback, confrontation, and process observation and feedback—may be distinguished. Each calls for special kinds of skills on the part of the consultant. For clients, it often is easier to classify these types of interventions simply into training and consultation and then to contrast the highly structured pedagogical formats of training with the more immediately pragmatic features of data feedback, confrontation, and process observation and feedback. Illustrations of each of the macrodesigns can be found in Schmuck, Runkel, Arends, and Arends (1977).

In training, the system-process consultant determines the learning goals for a scheduled time period, initiates structure, and directs activities. Training involves highly planned teaching and experience-based learning in structured formats that usually include lectures and assigned readings. It is similar in its procedures to traditional classroom teaching, except that in system-process consultation the key members of a subsystem or of an entire organization experience the training simultaneously and with one another. The training activities may include skills, exercises, and practice with procedures. Skills denote ways in which interactions can be executed within a group. They are put to work only in reciprocal relations among persons; no individual can make use of them in isolation. An exercise, or simulation, is a structured, gamelike activity designed to make prominent certain types of group processes that participants can easily conceptualize because they are related to their personal experience. Unlike exercises, whose content is determined by the consultant, procedures are content-free and are used for the purpose of making work more effective toward whatever goal has been chosen.

Data feedback, the systematic collecting of information that is tactfully reported back to key members of appropriate subsystems as a basis for diagnosis, is one of the most important intervention modes of the system-process consultant. At least three aspects of a data feedback strategy seem to constitute the keys of its success. First, the consultant must be adept at collecting valid, relevant data and at putting the data into feedback formats that will be understandable and motivating to the participants. Second, the consultant must strive to elevate mundane data to a level of larger, essential significance so that the data are worthy of notice by the participants. Third, the consultant must find ways of incorporating data feedback into the ebb and flow of larger consultative designs and should look for opportunities to transfer the task of data collection and feedback from the change project to the formal organization itself.

A confrontation design aims at publicly specifying the character of the social relationship between two or more role takers or subsystems, as well as at specifying the problems that are contributing to conflicts among them. The system-process consultant brings two (or more) bodies together to interact and to share the perceptions that each has of the other, to identify areas where each is viewed as helpful or unhelpful to the other, to establish clear communication channels between the two groups, to introduce a problem-solving procedure that may facilitate collaborative inquiry into mutual problems, and finally to specify the common concerns that cut across all parties involved in the confrontation.

In executing process observation and feedback, the purpose of which is to help group members become more aware of how they are working together, the system-process consultant sits with the client group during its work sessions, observes the ongoing processes, and occasionally offers personal comments or observations. This type of intervention aims to involve the participants in analyzing their working relationships and in making group agreements to modify the ways in which they will work together.

Training, data feedback, confrontation, and process observation and feedback each in a different way sets the stage for collaborative problem solving, plan making, and experimental trials. Although in reality the four types of intervention are often incorporated into a single macrodesign for system improvement in a complex organization, Figure 5-3 summarizes the point of emphasis of each in relation to the consultant's targets for improving system health.

Figure 3

Typical Emphases (/) Among Targets of System Health and Intervention Designs

	Train-ing	Data feed-back	Confron-tation	Process observa-tion and feedback
Interpersonal Skills				
Process information	✓	✓		
Problem identification	✓	✓		
Taking experimental action	✓	✓		✓
Subsystem Norms and Roles (within)				
Communication	✓	✓		✓
Goal setting	✓	✓		✓
Conflict management	✓	✓		✓
Meetings	✓	✓		✓
Problem solving	✓	✓		✓
Decision making	✓	✓		✓
Subsystem Norms and Roles (between)				
Communication	✓	✓	✓	✓
Goal setting	✓	✓	✓	✓
Conflict management	✓	✓	✓	✓
Meetings	✓	✓	✓	✓
Problem solving	✓	✓	✓	✓
Decision making	✓	✓	✓	✓
System Capacity for Problem Solving				
Systematic diagnosis		✓		✓
Proactive retrieval				✓
Cross-subsystem action planning			✓	✓
Self-analytic evaluation		✓	✓	✓

Summary

Many mental health difficulties arise out of people's participation in unhealthy social systems. The primary characteristics of a social system are its formal and informal norms, structures, and procedures that are organized by its generic subsystems, each concerned with production, support, maintenance, adaptation, and management. Healthy systems have participants who are self-actualizing through the satisfaction of their achievement, power, and affiliation strivings; subsystems with high productivity and a high quality of life; and an organizational capacity to solve system problems continuously. The system-process consultant enhances system health by upgrading interpersonal skills, by refurbishing subsystem norms and roles, and by developing a capacity within the entire social system for problem solving. The last involves facilitating development of formal norms, structures, and procedures that support systematic diagnosis; proactive retrieval of needed resources; cross-subsystem action planning; and self-analytic evaluation. Four strategies for intervening to improve the health of social system processes include training, data feedback, confrontation, and process observation and feedback.

References

Berlew, D. Leadership and Organizational Excitement. In D. A. Kolb, I. M. Rubin, & J. M. McIntyre (Eds.), *Organizational psychology: A book of readings* (2nd ed.). Englewood Cliffs, N.J.: Prentice-Hall, 1974, pp. 265-277.

Buckley, W. Sociology and modern systems theory. Englewood Cliffs, N.J.: Prentice-Hall, 1967.

Katz, D., & Kahn, R. *Social psychology of organizations* (2nd ed.). New York: Wiley, 1978.

McClelland, D. Methods of measuring human motivation. In J. W. Atkinson (Ed.), *Motives in fantasy, action, and society.* New York: Van Nostrand, 1958, pp. 7-42.

Miller, J. G. *Living systems.* New York: McGraw-Hill, 1978.

Osgood, C., & Suci, G. Factor analysis of meaning. *Journal of Experimental Psychology,* 1955, *50,* 325-338.

Schmuck, R., Runkel, P., Arends, J., & Arends, R. *The second handbook of organization development in schools.* Palo Alto, Calif.: Mayfield, 1977.

Part III

ISSUES

Chapter 6

ISSUES IN CONSULTATION

Saul Cooper, M.A.
William F. Hodges, Ph.D.

Much of the content of the following four chapters relates to issues of tech-nique and skill in carrying out consultation. There is an implied assump-tion about a stable parent organization. All too often the aspiring con-sultant launches bravely into other organizations and systems, with high motivation and, it is hoped, some beginning skills. This launching forth may from the outset be a high-risk activity if the consultant has not care-fully prepared her or his own agency linkages to support external activities.

GOALS

We frequently find a lack of congruence around both values and goals between the consultant's parent organization and the consultant himself or herself. Since consultants often find themselves with very little power in their own systems, they tend to focus much of their energy on external behaviors rather than facing the most difficult issues endemic to their own system. This inner-directed organizational perspective is a continuous maintenance activity that cannot be ignored, however. Every effective con-sultant must develop a strategy for dealing with value and goal discrepancies within his or her own organization or the entire consultation program will always be at great risk.

One finds, for example, that directors of mental health centers frequently translate values and goals directly into a high priority for clinical intervention. This translation is neither necessary nor inevitable, and there are opportunities for an effective consultant to make clear how consultation intervention might equally fulfill the values and goals espoused by the director or by the board of the mental health organization.

Careful planning of a community intervention requires the best skills of the consultant. Data gathering, diagnosing, and designing of community consultation programs take considerable time and energy. No less than this should be expected of the consultant in relation to one's own agency.

MODELS

There are a variety of ways of reflecting values. Service delivery models, including how one develops the organizational structure of consultation services within the parent organization, are one way that values are reflected.

Three organizational models for consultation are offered here: (1) the specialist model, (2) the generalist model, and (3) the matrix model. Although these models will be discussed in relation to mental health consultation, they are equally relevant for mental health center organization generally. Each model implies a value frame, and in many centers, the experience and training of the staff tends to lead to a model. Inferences about values can be drawn, but are not made explicit as often as they should be. The degree of consonance between the mental health center organizational model and the consultation organizational model in any given setting will have a great deal to do with the quality and amount of mental health consultation delivered.

The specialist model might be described as function specific but administratively isolated. In this model, if the director of consultation services designs an organizational structure that takes into account only the needs relating to external delivery of consultation services, and if that structure is not compatible with the remainder of the structure of the mental health center, then one actually has visible evidence of a discrepancy between values.

In the generalist model, a middle-level management team influences policy and programming in a significant way. Let us posit that the director of consultation services is not part of that middle-management team, but rather deals directly with the chief executive officer of the mental health center. On the face of it, this direct-line link from the consultation director to the mental health center director might seem to be a distinct advantage, but, over time, this organizational pattern will further isolate consultation services from the mainstream of clinical activities at the center, ultimately increasing the risk and the credibility problems of the consultation service.

In the specialist model, where there are a small number of highly specialized consultants, the greatest danger appears to be almost total isolation and ultimate alienation from the rest of the staff and administrators of the mental health center. On the one hand, it is a highly attractive model for service delivery since it minimizes coordination problems and maximizes skill development in a small number of people. On the other hand, this distancing produces obvious risks when a scarcity of resources occurs. Unless consultation programs can be assured of independent funding or can be maintained through reimbursement for services, one should not be too optimistic about the long-term viability of a consultation program built entirely around a specialist model.

The generalist model, with one consultation coordinator and a sizable number of part-time consultants who are for the most part clinicians, produces a different set of problems. Primarily one finds in such a situation that consultation services are most at risk when emergency demands are placed on clinicians. Given the high demand for clinical services and some degree of unpredictability of emergencies, one finds that clinicians set aside their consultation obligations when stress of this sort occurs. Further, one finds that design and orchestration of an agencywide consultation program are extremely difficult to bring about with a large number of part-time consultants. Each consultant tends to have an area of special interest or concern and would much prefer to be left alone to carry out this type of consultation without being heavily involved in an agencywide commitment.

The weaknesses of such a model are obvious, but the strengths are not quite so obvious. One strength is that survival of consultation services is much more likely with this type of generalist model than with the specialist model. Clinicians tend to value the "change of pace" of doing consultation. It serves as a respite from hour-by-hour clinical practice. To the extent that such values exist in a mental health center, clinicians who are part-time consultants will tend to support the ongoing need for a consultation program. A further point to be emphasized has both a negative and a positive quality to it, and that is the notion that all clinicians can do consultation, since consultation is little more than an extension of clinical practice in the community. The negative aspect of this attitude is that clinicians-turned-consultants can carry out extremely poor and sometimes even destructive consultation activities in the community. The positive aspect of this perception is that consultation is not a unique and totally separate type of service, but in fact fits into the normal activities of the staff members of the mental health center.

In our experience, the most organizationally stable consultation programs are those that are administratively designed to be highly consonant with the values and goals of the director and the board of the mental health center. Neither a generalist nor a specialist model has intrinsic value: they must be assessed within the organizational context of the parent agency. It appears that a matrix model embedded in the organizational mainstream of a mental health center is most highly correlated with successful programs.

Up to this point, we have addressed organizational issues from a mental health center perspective. Let us now turn to the consultant who uses a university setting as an organizational base.

Entry issues frequently revolve around the academician-consultant being perceived as a researcher or a trainer of students. In either case, these role perceptions frequently have other motives attached to them. If there is any question about a hidden agenda, it should be dealt with early, frequently, and honestly. Although agencies and consultees will often accept students as consultants, this assumption should be tested at entry. Nor can one assume a set of dynamics in which faculty will always be preferable to students. Trust issues at entry are one of the earliest hurdles that need to be addressed.

Another issue faced by the academician-consultant is similar to one already identified in the case of a mental health center. How is consultation defined by the consultant to the university? Is it a contributed community service activity? Is it an opportunity to gather teaching-training materials? Is it a paid private practice arrangement? Does the consultee system ever deal directly with the academician-consultant's parent organization, the university? The organizational context of an academician-consultant has rarely been addressed in the literature, and we would urge our colleagues to begin to deal with it.

TRAINING ISSUES

Special issues related to student training can be found in mental health centers as well as universities. We frequently find a student assigned to consultation services for one or two semesters, at which point a new student comes along to attempt to move in where the previous student left off. In effect, over a 5-year period one could deliver 5 years of consultation, but it would have been made up of anywhere from 5 to 10 students. The incremental value of this type of staffing pattern is highly questionable. It has been our experience that 5 years worth of anywhere from 5 to 10 consultants may, in a very crude way, add up to about a half year of progress with a given consultee system. We find that consultee systems are as much impressed by the individual consultant and the trust relationship built up with him or her as they are with the actual consultation activities being delivered. In fact, after working with a highly successful, empathic student consultant, consultees are often unwilling or reluctant even to try to build trust with someone new.

After an experience with an ineffective student consultant, reentry will, of course, be difficult. This attributed trust or credibility in individuals is extremely difficult to overcome, and when programming with difficult systems, the consultation team should keep in mind that more permanent staffing patterns are more likely to produce significant progress over time. Specifically, if one estimates a 3- to 5-year commitment with a particular system, such as a sheriff's department, in order to produce the type of program and organizational changes necessary, then it would be inadvisable to use student resources as the major staffing pattern.

We do find that one can carry out a successful consultation program within an extensive student training program; but in order to do so, the consultant supervisor must commit a significant amount of time to consultee-system maintenance. The ongoing trust and linkages must be built between the consultant supervisor and the consultee system. Short-term students are not likely to carry out such a task successfully.

Issues of records, confidentiality, malpractice, and fees are even more complex when the bulk of the consultation service is being delivered by students.

CONSULTATION ISSUES: AN OVERVIEW

The Mann chapter attempts to lay out some of the context and specific activities involved in mental health consultation. One needs to stress the ecological perspective in all these activities.

One can conceive of issues that are related to the provider agency, that is, the mental health center itself; issues related to the consumer agency; and finally issues related to the community in which both the provider and the consumer agency exist. This systemic contextual approach to consultation is extremely important if one is to develop and strengthen consultation programming over time.

Perhaps the most frequent topic of conversation when consultants come together is economics and accountability in consultation. The Shore and Mannino chapter attempts to highlight some of the issues involved. There are creative approaches one can consider around the economics of consultation services. One can arrange a "bartering" between the consultant agency and the consultee agency. A school system that has a media specialist on staff might well trade some hours of service from the media specialist for consultation services. The media specialist could be extremely helpful to the mental health center in designing community relations activities or preparing reports for the board or for other funding agencies.

One might barter client transportation to inpatient facilities with the sheriff's department, or one could trade home visits for consultation with a nursing group. Bartering cannot pay staff salaries and overhead, but it not only represents "income" to the mental health center, perhaps more important it reflects the fact that a value has been placed on the service not only by the consultant but also by the consultee. We suspect that a number of rather innovative approaches to bartering could easily be developed in mental health centers around the country.

In the realm of innovations one should also consider a distinction between charging for all consultation services and billing for all consultation services. It would appear that many consultee agencies cannot or will not pay for services and therefore would not agree to receive a bill for such activities. Sometimes one can enter into an understanding with the consultee agency which allows the consulting agency to charge for services rendered. Such a charge might well be in the form of a bill, but there would be an understanding that payment is not expected, at least not in the early stages of a consultation program. The existence of a charge communicates to the consultee agency rather clearly both the amount and the actual cost of the services delivered. It also allows the consulting agency to maintain a systematic and visible record of not only the amount of effort but also the amount of dollars expended in carrying out that effort.

This model for charging follows very closely the typical practices of clinical services, in which there is either a partial or a full writeoff depending upon the circumstances of the client. As described in the Shore and Mannino chapter, accountability in consultation demands a clear set of agreed-upon definitions and standards for services. Some mental health centers have no record-keeping system and certainly no definitions and standards; other centers have a unique "homegrown" model for both record keeping and standards. In neither case can accountability be adequately managed. Two efforts currently under way would seem to be addressing this issue. The Southern Regional Education Board, under Dr. Harold McPheeters, is working to develop definitions of prevention services. The Prevention Council of the National Council of Community Mental Health Centers had a task force which recently completed a similar project. In the final analysis, the field of mental health consultation cannot hope to move ahead without a minimal set of definitions and standards.

The other aspect of accountability, namely, a management information system, has also been addressed on an agency-by-agency basis. There is no doubt that survival and credibility for consultation within one's own agency are highly dependent upon such a management information system. If the procedures and definitions of the consultation service are totally idiosyncratic in relation to other procedures and definitions in the overall management information system of the agency, then problems are likely to arise. It is strongly advised that the consultation unit attempt to produce as much compatibility as possible with the existing management information system of its own agency. Here again, in the absence of state or national standards, each local consultation program should have an accountability system that best fits its own agency. Whatever the data-generating capacity, the parent agency should at the very least have a data system for consultation equal to its data system for clinical services.

One of the more insidious problems in this general area of economics and accountability has to do with the delicate balance of income and relevance. One can guarantee sufficient income for a consultation program by large ignoring the true mental health needs of a community. This leads to what can be called "macrame for mental health," that is, offering programs and services that are guaranteed to generate income but which have little demonstrable relationship to the major service needs in a community. Good consultation programming requires a balance between programming for income and programming for need. Maintaining that balance is one of the most important challenges facing mental health consultants at the moment. We would much prefer to see this balance addressed honestly rather than seeing elaborate need justification developed to defend a program built for income. Unfortunately the needs for consultation in a community rarely coincide with the dollars available to pay for such services.

Mental health professionals have always devoted some time to concerns around ethics and values. The Lippitt chapter attempts to lay out some notions that need to be addressed by consultation programs. When one considers the enormous complexity of the consultation process across systems, consultants, consultees, and clients, it becomes quite obvious that ethics and values as issues cannot be avoided.

Perhaps the most common issue in this category is confidentiality. We find a variety of problems barely being addressed that have to do with confidentiality among and between consultants, clients, and systems. In some mental health centers, standards developed for clinical practice are applied almost unheedingly to consultation practice. Are the same standards appropriate? Can they be applied in exactly the same way? What about records? Who owns a consultation record? How do we interpret informed consent in consultation? Although most of these issues are only occasionally discussed in the literature, all of them must be addressed by any responsible consultation program. A good consultation program will address these issues for itself in an explicit fashion and continue to work toward resolving the complexities that are brought up.

Kelly's chapter opens up issues related to the long-term goal of the consultant. In essence, to be effective one goes about eliminating the need for a consultant in the consultee agency. Kelly talks about the creation of power and some of the specific behaviors involved. In addition, one needs to consider the consequences for a consultant of creating power in a consultee system. Power is created for the consultee by increasing the consultee's ability to increase resources available to solve problems. Experienced consultants must recognize that creating power can be stressful for the consultant, who then may feel less powerful as a consultant. For competent professionals this should not be an issue; for beginning consultants who need reinforcement and gratification, creating power in consultee systems may be antithetical to their own needs. At the very least, the mental health center must be sensitive to the positive-reinforcement requirements of all its consultants that will be necessary to free them up so they can work comfortably in creating power in consultee systems.

There is very little doubt that consultation as a technique will continue to exist in the field of mental health, but there is some doubt that consultation as an organized field of practice will continue to exist unless consultants address the issues identified in the following four chapters.

Chapter 7

TRANSITION POINTS IN CONSULTATION
ENTRY, TRANSFER, AND TERMINATION

Philip A. Mann, Ph.D.

Mental health consultation has been a required part of community mental health services since the initial federal legislation providing funding for community mental health centers (CMHCs) was passed. Yet it has remained the least well developed and least understood of the required CMHC services. Among the many reasons for this state of affairs, one is the fact that most CMHC personnel take an individual, intrapsychic approach to their work with clients or patients. This perspective has limited generalizability to the work of consultation. The topics of entry, transfer, and termination, to be discussed in this chapter, especially require a focus on the level of social systems rather than on individuals. Another limitation is imposed in the form of low demand for consultation services from community agencies. No doubt the frequent expectation of consultees for direct services rather than consultation is based on a perception of CMHC personnel expertise as limited to individual intrapsychic problems, a perception that is all too often an accurate one.

Consultation has the potential to be a strategy aimed at prevention, to compensate for the limited supply of mental health professionals, and to enhance the help-giving capacity of natural care givers. It is important that community mental health services define and make visible consultation as a problem-solving process available to consultee systems in the community. In turn, it is essential that consultants understand the consulting task as helping community organizations to (1) solve their problems, (2) become self-sufficient, and (3) adapt to future needs, in enhancing the mental health of the organization's clients.

Within this problem-solving process, entry, transfer, and termination are important transition points. Understanding of the problems associated with each of these points is necessary to effective consultation, but these understandings by themselves are not sufficient for planning a consultation program, as other chapters in this volume indicate. Examination of entry, transfer, and termination questions can be helpful in starting a consultation program, and, as with all other aspects of the consultation process, this examination should be undertaken before consultation is begun. Such considerations include what have been called preentry issues, and these issues form a beginning point for this discussion.

PREENTRY ISSUES

When presented with an opportunity for consultation, the consultant must consider a number of questions in planning one's approach to the consultee system. Cherniss (1976) labeled this cluster of questions *preentry* issues. The first question to be entertained is whether or not consultation should be undertaken. It may be that alternative interventions will be more appropriate or more effective than consultation, or that no intervention by the consultant or the consultant's agency should be made around a particular problem. Among the considerations bearing on this question are the value congruencies between the consultants and the consultee system, the resources available for bringing about change, the characteristics of potential consultees, and the influence of the social milieu.

Consideration of these issues may present a dilemma for the would-be consultant who is attempting to develop a consultation program and create visibility for consultation activities. Under these conditions, the consultant may be inclined to accept whatever opportunities arise. It is well, however, to remember that inappropriate or ineffective consultation may be worse than none at all in meeting these goals. At this level, the question is not whether consultation can be done, but whether consultation is the most appropriate approach to the problem.

Some would-be consultants incorrectly see consultation as a method of reform. Accordingly these consultants may seek to establish consultation relationships with such public institutions as police or schools in order to correct what they see as deficiencies in these systems, a view that is not likely to be shared by the members of police departments or school faculties. Conversely, legitimate requests for consultation from such institutions may be declined by consultants who disagree with what they see as the dominant values or goals of these organizations. This is clearly the case in the attitude of many consultants toward police departments.[1] Congruence of values, goals, and expectations is considered an important prerequisite to consultation (Glidewell, 1959; Levine, 1970), and there is some evidence that it is related to consultation outcome (Mann, 1973a). If congruent values do not exist *or cannot be discovered or created,* consultants may do well to decline to enter such consultation relationships.

Lippitt (1959) included among the questions that should guide beginning consultation whether the consultant has the resources required for bringing about necessary changes in a consultee system. These resources include both time and skill. It will often happen that a consultee system will overestimate a consultant's resources, tending to generate unrealistically high expectations. On the other side of this question is the time for making members of the consultee system available for consultation. This is a frequent problem in consulting with police, whose "down time," when they might be available for consultation, occurs out in the field rather than at a central location. Similarly, teachers will have to have free time away from classrooms to meet with the consultant. In consultee systems with heavy task demands, this resource may not be readily available. An important question, then, is whether task requirements can be modified to create this needed resource.

Assessing whether potential consultees have whatever characteristics may be required for successful consultation is difficult to accomplish at a distance, since consultants' stereotypes may enter into the process. Accordingly some reconnaissance of the consultee system may be needed in the form of preliminary meetings or discussions. Occasionally the consultant may be well enough acquainted with members of the consultee system to make this determination without further acquaintance. Care should be taken, however, to distinguish between what the consultant thinks the consultees *ought* to be able to do and what they are actually capable of doing.

Requests for consultation are sometimes generated from requirements in consultee systems, rather than from a perceived need for change within the system itself; for example, federal guidelines for such programs as Head Start and the Job Corps have required the use of mental health consultants, but personnel in these programs sometimes have only a vague idea of what consultation is and often do not see a need for change or development within their own organization. I was once approached by the leaders of one such program with a request for consultation because they had been told by a federal evaluator to obtain such help. It became apparent that what they wanted was someone to screen out those students who did not conform to the program on grounds of psychopathology, and I declined the request when the organization expressed uninterest in consultee- or program-centered consultation. Requests for direct clinical services are frequently guised as requests for consultation under such circumstances, and a careful evaluation of the needs behind such requests will usually indicate the most appropriate response. As Caplan said concerning consultation with many newly formed organizations, "They ask for a consultant, but they need someone who will combine consultation with straightforward teaching, supervision, and collaboration—someone who will 'pitch in and get his hands dirty'" (Caplan, 1970, p. xii). In assessing such requests, the consultant must determine if the resources for meeting the immediate problem are available and whether such a relationship can provide access to a future role that might address questions that would be appropriate for consultative intervention.

Another question concerning consultation raised by Cherniss is the question of whose interests are to be served. Consultants may expect to be approached at times by organizations that are under fire of public criticism, and the consultant will want to determine that the consultation is sought for more than just cosmetic reasons. The question of what constituency will ultimately benefit from the consultation effort has an important bearing on the resolution of this issue. Multiple interest groups make demands of service organizations, especially public institutions. Psychologists may undertake consultation with police departments because of the strategic role of the police in handling mental health problems, only to find that various interest groups have competing expectations concerning the effects of such work on police-community relations. Some community members may expect that such efforts will produce more responsive and sensitive police behavior toward minority groups, while others, including the police themselves, may see consultation as an effort to improve the professional image of the police in the interest of supporting demands for higher pay. In school settings, consultation may be sought in order to sanction efforts at increased behavioral control and exclusion of disruptive students on mental health grounds when, in fact, the rigidity of the school social system may generate an excessive number of cases of disruption.

At a minimum, it is important to clarify and make visible the appropriate expectations for consultative intervention on the part of both consultant and consultees. Congruency of expectations is a desirable prerequisite to consultation, but it is also desirable that members of the consultee system have the potential to see the relationships among their own needs, those of their constituencies, and any planned changes in the consultee system.

Assuming that these issues are resolved in the direction of beginning consultation with a social system, further planning of the actual consultative effort is in order. Many of the concerns relative to this process were outlined by Lippitt (1959). These include an assessment of the consultant's motives for working with the consultee system and of the motivations

within the consultee system for and against change. Requests for consultation will usually include a suggested goal for the work, but it is important
for the consultant to clarify for himself or herself both what the focus of the
consultation will be and how the proposed method of work is related to the
expected outcome. Often this relationship is based on a number of assumptions that require critical examination. Will changes in individuals result in
changes in the structure of the consultee system, if that is what is needed? If
such individual changes are achieved, will the consultee system or its social
environment be able to sustain them? At this point, it is often helpful, if not
necessary, to introduce the role of evaluation. If the desired changes are
achieved, how will anyone know? Are the desired outcomes measurable in
any way, and is it reasonable to expect that the measures that might be
employed will truly reflect the desired changes? Answers to these questions
may be suggested by examining both the consultant's and the consultee
system's previous experience with similar change efforts, as well as theories
and techniques applicable to the particular set of problems to be addressed.

A final note concerning preentry issues is in order. Many consultants
operate on what is a reactive model; that is, they respond to requests for
consultation services as they are received. But persons in settings with
communitywide responsibilities, such as CMHCs, may wish to take the
initiative in approaching some key community organizations, such as
schools, police, or courts, to discuss intervention programs that may have
primary or secondary preventive goals. Such undertakings magnify both
the preentry issues and the problems associated with the entry process itself,
but they do not alter the basic principles involved. Approaching such
organizations with preconceived intervention programs, including consultation, would be obviously premature and likely to generate resistance, if
not rejection.

A sound strategy was suggested by Caplan (1970, pp. 35-47), based on
an assessment of the community's history, needs, and resources. The key
ingredients of this approach are to make contact and develop relationships
with a wide range of community agencies. These steps may be taken as part
of the assessment process initially, and may progress to collaborative
activities other than consultation that foster relationship building. The
importance of establishing these relationships and, to use Caplan's term,
"creating proximity" to key community institutions cannot be overstated
and may prove invaluable when opportunities arise for consultation,
especially during periods of crisis, when time does not permit relationship
building but requires action (Mann & Iscoe, 1971). In many ways, these
processes merely duplicate the activities that must be conducted anyway
during the entry stage of consultation.

ENTRY

The entry stage can be described as a process through which the consultant becomes temporarily attached to a social system (Glidewell, 1959). The nature of this relationship is at once advantageous and problematic. As an outsider, the consultant enjoys a certain freedom from role constraints that is not available to regular members of the system, allowing her or him to suggest innovative actions and to relate to persons across the structure of the consultee system. At the same time, the consultant wants to achieve understanding and acceptance of role functions within the organization. These two goals are potentially conflicting, the more so in highly structured consultee systems, and tend to create ambiguity for potential consultees.

Members of the consultee system may vary in their approach to the consultant because of the tension between acceptance of the consultant and the consultant's status as an outsider. The following example illustrates this tension. While a consultant was riding on patrol with a police officer in order to become familiar with police operations, the officer gave a motorist a ticket for speeding. Later the officer asked the consultant if he would be willing to appear as a witness in case the motorist contested the citation. The consultant declined, on the grounds that it would confuse the definition of his role as a consultant, but used the opportunity to sympathize with the officer's frustration over having to deal with such resistance. (The motorist was clearly speeding.) The consultant wanted to separate his role from the law enforcement function, but also did not want to appear distant and uninvolved with the officer's concerns. One of the consultant's tasks is to maintain a creative tension between these goals so as to achieve the optimal amount of both freedom and acceptance that will facilitate the consultant's acting as an agent of change. In this sense, then, the entry stage may be said to continue throughout the consultation, although at differing levels of the consultee system.

Accordingly the consultant's first concern is making contact with and gaining access to the consultee system. If it has not been the point of first contact, the consultant will want to meet with members of the highest administrative level of the system to obtain sanction for working with the organization and to clarify expectations of the consultant's role. Depending on previous relationships between the consultant's own organization and the consultee system, this meeting may include top administrative staff from the consultant's agency as well. The latter step may be particularly helpful with status-conscious administrators who may otherwise "go over the consultant's head" in reporting perceived problems to the consultant's administrator rather than to the consultant or who may feel that the consultant is there to serve the rest of the organization but not the top administration.

In addition to discussing the aims and scope of the consultation, those present at this meeting should arrange for the consultant to meet with the other members of the consultee system. The availability of the consultant and of potential consultees needs to be made explicit, and some means of scheduling meetings with the consultant should be agreed upon. Trivial though it may seem, more than one consultant has shown up expecting to meet with consultees, only to find that none were available because of scheduling conflicts.

In negotiating these arrangements, the consultant must be sure that he or she has the commitment and support of his or her own agency for entering and maintaining the consultation relationship. Consultation services provided by CMHC staff members are rarely supported by fees, and without the CMHC's commitment to the consultation, a change in funding or in service priorities may necessitate a reduction or termination of the consultation relationship. Such an eventuality can be damaging to the relationships of both the consultant and the CMHC to community agencies and conceivably could affect adversely the agencies' willingness to make referrals as well as attitudes toward future consulting arrangements.

The initial contacts with the consultee system provide a basis for the task of familiarization (Jarvis & Nelson, 1967). This process can be vital to the consultant's learning not only the usual practices of consultees in performing their duties, but also the constraints that operate on alternative activities. In the absence of the familiarization task, consultants might work to bring about changes in the activities of consultees that are limited by social forces or legal requirements. The danger is not so much that consultees will implement inappropriate changes as it is that the consultant's efforts will encounter legitimate resistance and the effort will be wasted, if not counterproductive, that is, these efforts may mobilize resistance against legitimate change. In effect, this problem is a particular case of Lippitt's prescription (1959) that the consultant should assess the forces for and against change.

The familiarization task may be critical for assessing and managing resistance forces, an obstacle that the consultant must always anticipate. Some of these forces are systemic in nature. Any social system must contain substantial forces that are resistant to change in order for that system to maintain any degree of stability (Katz & Kahn, 1966). Other types of resistance may stem from individual attitudes and beliefs or from the position of certain individuals in relation to the social system. Mann (1972), for example, found that there was an inverse relationship between the accessibility to a consultant of components of an organization and the standing of those components in the organization's power structure. Organizational components with less social power were more accessible than those with more social power. Hirschman (1974) found that this relationship held for individual consultees as well.

The consultant who takes a social system perspective can anticipate and recognize different kinds of resistance and can learn to distinguish between the systemic and personal forms of resistance. This kind of information can be invaluable in planning consultative interventions. Otherwise the perceptions and attitudes of persons who are marginal in the power structure of the consultee system may be mistakenly seen as characteristic of the entire system, and the consultant who proceeds to act accordingly may find that she or he is in a position of advocating change that has little centrality to the system or is seen as a socializing agent for marginal elements of the system with no influence on the more essential workings of the consultee system. If the consultant should act on this initial information, attempts to produce changes may instead mobilize increased resistance. Awareness of these phenomena of social system workings can alert the consultant to determine how widely shared are perceptions of problems and orientations toward change within the organization.

The familiarization task also has reciprocal aspects for potential consultees. As an outsider, the consultant represents an unfamiliar object for members of the consultee system, and the familiarization process is an opportunity for them to become better acquainted with both the role and the personality of the consultant. Many consultees will overvalue the status, power, and expertise of the consultant. Interaction during the familiarization task can be used to work toward establishing the kind of coordinate relationship that consultation requires (Caplan, 1970), if the consultant takes the stance of a learner toward the work of the consultee. By taking this position, the consultant communicates that he or she regards the consultee as competent and knowledgeable in the latter's field and that the consultant's own professional expertise is not in competition with that of the consultee. Sarason et al. (1966) introduced themselves as consultants to teachers with the pointed comment that they appreciated the difficulties of the teacher's roles, respected the competencies that those roles required, and themselves had no desire to change places with the teachers.

In spite of this effort, two additional problems arise often enough to require further comments. One of these is the persistence of the myth that the consultant really does have the definitive answer to the consultee's problems, and that if the consultant would just reveal this magical truth, the consultee and consultant could both save a lot of time and trouble. The consultant who is seduced by this kind of flattering expectation, which is at best an ambivalent expectation on the part of the consultee (who is both wanting an answer and being afraid that answers would prove his or her own incompetence), is treading on very thin ice. The consultant can avoid this trap if he or she regards both the impressions gained during the familiarization process and any possible interventions as tentative, as hypotheses to be examined more fully and tested in subsequent work. By being willing to learn from consultees and assuming an initial stance somewhat analogous to the one that a cultural anthropologist might take toward a native guide, the consultant can gain valuable information, diminish some of the threat that consultees may feel, and define the consultant's role as one that avoids premature conclusions based on inadequate information.

The second problem is the stereotype that attaches to the helping professions, which may lead the consultee to the wish, the fear, or both that the consultant will provide psychotherapy for the consultee's problems. Here it is important that the consultant clarify that the consulting role is confined to helping with the work-role-related problems of the consultee. Since the consultant cannot ordinarily determine immediately whether these requests for psychotherapy are genuine or are a way of testing the consultant's intentions, the consultant will do well to listen to such remarks as a sympathetic friend, but to avoid taking the stance of a therapist or diagnostician toward them. Sofer (1961) recommended that the consultant respond to consultees' raising personal problems by relating some similar personal difficulty that the consultant has experienced, thus putting consultant and consultee on a more equal footing and allowing the expression of sympathy and concern without accepting the problem as a psychotherapeutic possibility for the consultant. Should it develop that the problem is one that interferes with the consultee's work, Caplan (1970) recommended that the consultant may assist in referring the consultee to a psychotherapist, but that consultants should decline to enter a psychotherapeutic relationship with consultees because of the role confusions and personal threats that could arise throughout the consultee system from such a response.

Finally, an essential part of the familiarization task is to determine what problem-solving efforts have been attempted in the past, what degree of success they have achieved, and, where possible, the reasons for failure of the unsuccessful efforts. Not only does this step ensure the consultant against suggesting efforts that have already been disproven in the eyes of consultees, but also it helps to define consultees as problem solvers who have ideas of their own and to identify strengths and weaknesses in the problem-solving resources of the consultee system.

Although familiarization may continue throughout the consultation, the initial familiarization activity should culminate in a contract for implementation of consultative activity between the consultant and the consultee system. The contract, which should be discussed with members of the consultee system and then put into written form, will specify the method and timing of work, including arrangements for contact between consultant and consultees; the timing and nature of any data to be collected; and the expectations for and methods of accountability of the consultant to the consultee system. Data collection is often resisted, but is an important and indispensable procedure for meaningful consultation. Besides the data's being essential to subsequent evaluation of the consultation effort, a discussion of the kinds of data needed and the manner in which they might be collected can help to clarify and concretize the goals of consultation and can increase the awareness of consultant and consultees that those goals are shared. I have found it useful to include in the contract a provision for periodic review of the consultation with members of the consultee system and the possibility of modifying the contract as indicated by subsequent experience (Mann, 1973b). Here again, data collection can be useful in pointing out the need for, and possible directions of, modifications in the contract.

The term *contract* is used to denote a variety of meanings in professional services. In consultation relationships, the contract usually takes the form of an exchange of letters between the consultant and the consultee system, spelling out the expectations and obligations of each party, the frequency of meetings, the scheduling of appointments and access to personnel in the consultee system, the data to be collected, the provisions for review and modification of the program, and the amount and manner of payment of any fees involved. This exchange of letters is usually initiated by the consultant, who invites the administrator of the consultee system to reply. At times contracts may be more formal when fees are involved, depending upon the requirements of the consultee system or of a funding agency. The major advantage of a written contract that includes plans and expectations, over and above service and fee agreements, is its usefulness as a reference point for future review and evaluation and as a framework for definition of the consultant's role.

Consultants vary in the attention they give to value issues in consultation. Value issues may arise in a request for the consultant's services that violates in some way the consultant's values, in the discovery by the consultant of some organizational practice that is contrary to accepted social values, or in the form of consultees asking the consultant for a statement of her or his values on a controversial issue that may not be central to the consultative interaction. In consulting with a police organization, Monahan (Heller & Monahan, 1977) took care to state explicitly to the chief of police what his position was on a variety of value issues and the actions that he would take should these issues arise, prior to beginning the consultation. Thus these issues would be stated as part of the consultation contract.

The consultant's social responsibility when confronted with organizational practices that he or she views as inimical to human welfare is a thorny issue. Making such practices public will almost certainly jeopardize the consulting relationship, whereas remaining silent may be to abdicate social and ethical responsibility. The American Psychological Association task force on ethical issues for psychologists working with the criminal justice system debated this issue at length without satisfactory resolution.[2] The question is certainly not limited to police organizations. In practice, such instances are infrequent, but when they occur, the consultant brings the problem to the consultee system for discussion, and if the consultee system is unresponsive, the consultant may decide to terminate the relationship on ethical grounds. In discussing consulting with police organizations, the APA task force raised the question of whether the principle of confidentiality applies to consultants working with organizations in the same way that it does for psychologists working with individual clients. The ethical implications of this question have not been resolved, but experience indicates that the practical consequences of violating confidentiality would be to severely restrict opportunities for consultation.

When consultees solicit the consultant's personal opinion on value issues, it is important that the consultant separate his or her personal opinions about such issues from his or her role as a consultant, especially where the value issues are not central to the consultation activity. Solicitations of this kind may serve the consultee's wish to draw the consultant into revealing more of his or her personality, as if the consultant's value positions were important to a satisfactory working relationship. This consultee behavior may be a kind of "love me, love my dog" testing of the consultant's potential to satisfy consultee needs that are not central or appropriate to the consultation, or it may be a way of testing whether the consultant will intrude personal values into the working relationship. In either case, the consultant may respond to such questions by making an explicit statement that the opinion expressed is personal rather than professional. By demonstrating this separation, the consultant may set a useful example for the consultees in making such distinctions for themselves.

Completion of the familiarization process and establishment of a contractual understanding with the consultee system do not complete the entry stage of consultation. Entry is completed by the transition from the familiarization process to the implementation stage, a transition that involves the consultant's coming into contact with consultees in a working relationship. This passage is also marked by the overcoming of systemic resistance to the attachment of the consultant to the social system.

In keeping with Caplan's view of consultation as a voluntary relationship, he assumed that consultees will seek out the consultant because they are experiencing a crisis with a particular client. Benjamin, using a theoretical model in which crisis was defined as high emotionality and low confidence, found only partial support for the crisis assumption. Those using consultation most often were high in emotionality, but were also high in confidence, contrary to the theoretical expectation.[3]

Accordingly the consultant can regard utilization of consultation on two levels. As individuals, those consultees who seek consultation because they are in crisis or inexperienced or both should be more amenable to change; but these same considerations suggest that the impact of consultation on the total consultee system may be limited unless the consultant can gain access to a larger segment of the members of the consultee system. The research reviewed here indicated that this larger impact will occur only as systemic resistances are overcome, the salience of consultation to the consultees' work role is demonstrated, and new problems are defined that are compelling for persons who initially are disinclined to use consultation. Such progress requires that the consultant be able to gain access to the entire consultee system, and it is with this in mind that consultants seek to make contact with all members of the system during familiarization and to repeat such contacts periodically.

The transition from familiarization to implementation is often marked by the emergence of an interesting phenomenon, the gatekeeper role. In Lewin's conception of the gatekeeper phenomenon (1951), this role is one that controls the social forces surrounding a gate section in a channel that gives access to the functioning of a social system. The purpose of the gatekeeper is to control access to the setting. In educational settings, the gatekeeper role is often occupied by a counselor whose functions are seen as similar to those of the consultant and who may feel a sense of competition with the consultant. In police organizations, the gatekeeper role frequently falls to a police-community relations officer, whose function is often seen as dealing with all outside forces. It is worth noting that both these roles are often seen as marginal within the social system.

In addition to whatever sense of threat or duplication the gatekeeper may perceive in the consultant, the appearance of the gatekeeper role also reveals something about the functional perceptions of the social system as a whole. In schools, this perception is the view that the system's problems are related to needed changes in their clientele, or students. In police organizations, the perception is that problems stem from needed changes in the public image of the police function. Both these views tend to represent resistance to the idea that change is needed within the social system, on the part of its members. Accordingly the gatekeeper role is a manifestation of systemic resistance that must be overcome if change is to occur at a social system level.

Because of their strategic position, gatekeepers can be important sources of information about, as well as access to, the social system. The consultant who encounters this phenomenon will do well to establish a relationship with the gatekeeper that is similar to the way the cultural anthropologist relates to a guide to the other members of a tribe or village. It is important to agree on a separation of functions and identities between the consultant and the gatekeeper, but it is also important for the consultant to afford the latter the respect and esteem that is due this guiding function. Burke found that, where the gatekeeper function occurs, the transition from entry to implementation is delayed, but overcoming this form of systemic resistance and turning it to consultative advantage is a necessary step in the transition process.[4]

Another approach is to schedule meetings with groups of consultees. These groups will have to be selected for their strategic significance in the makeup of the consultee system, according to patterns of communication and influence that exist. Group meetings may increase accessibility of individual consultees to the consultant, and individual consultation may provide information to the consultant that suggests a need for group meetings as several common or socially significant problems are identified. The consultant who can maintain flexibility in the matter of relating to the social system on several different levels can increase his or her usefulness in helping the consultee system to address and solve its problems.

To the extent that group consultation may be less voluntary on the part of the individual consultee than is one-to-one consultation, and particularly where group processes focus on the consultation method, the consultant will need to be especially sensitive to the coercive forces that may be set in motion. Since effective consultation is based on personal relationships and on referent power rather than coercive power (Bennis, 1966), this concern is a strategic as well as an ethical one.

Inasmuch as the consultant can expect to have to continue to define or redefine her or his role, many of the tasks involved in the entry stage will reoccur in implementing the planned consultation activity. In this sense the entry stage is never quite completed. The transition from entry to implementation, however, should be marked by an increase in problem-solving relationships and a corresponding decline in the need for consultant role definition. The discussion can now turn to another point of transition, the replacement of one consultant by another.

TRANSFER OF CONSULTANTS

Although consultation activity is ordinarily planned with the assumption that the consultant or consultants will remain with the consultee system until termination, the need to transfer responsibility from one consultant to another may still arise. Unplanned needs for transfer may arise when the original consultant is unable to continue because of a change in his or her employment or obligations prior to termination of the consultation. Another unplanned need for tranfer may occur when new problems emerge in the consultee system that require skills which can be provided better by another consultant than by the original one. Planned needs for transfer arise most often when a consulting relationship is used for training purposes and trainees are replaced at the end of their training period.

Transfer involves two processes: termination of the relationship with the original consultant, and entry into the system of the new consultant, both of which are discussed elsewhere in this paper. Although planned duration of consultation relationships may vary, termination is an eventuality to be addressed in all consulting relationships. In keeping with the aim of helping the consultee system to become self-sufficient in problem solving, the consultant seeks to avoid becoming indispensable to the consultee system throughout the relationship, by managing dependency expectations and encouraging consultee autonomy. At the same time, the consultant's attachment to the consultee system will have created a set of expectations that will unavoidably resist change during the transfer process. The new consultant has the disadvantage of comparison with the former consultant, but also has the advantage of a precedent of use of a helping agent by the consultee system.

The difficulty of transfer will also be affected by the stage of consultation in which it occurs. The need for transfer should be discussed openly with members of the consultee system. Assuming that a reasonable degree of congruency of expectations has been established between consultant and consultees, it will need to be made clear that the new consultant understands and accepts these expectations. If reasonably congruent expectations have not been developed, then transfer may intensify resistance problems that already exist. In either case, these difficulties can be addressed by use of the principle of contiguity. This can be done by planned overlap in the contact of the two consultants with the consultee system. By accompanying the original consultant, the new consultant has an opportunity to clarify with the former any questions that may arise concerning the consultation, as well as to be introduced to the consultee system and to make up ground lost by not being involved in the original entry process. This use of dual consultants for a period of time eases the transfer of consultees' relationships to the new consultant. In addition to establishment of effective working relationships, one measure of completion of the transfer process is when consultees address problems to the new consultant without reference to the former consultant.

The possible need to transfer consultants is one factor that makes the use of multiple consultants from the beginning advantageous. The author discussed elsewhere the benefits of use of a consultant group in working with a social system.[5] This model was originally developed as an aid to introducing graduate student interns to the consultation process, but it has other strategic advantages as well. The relationships with the consultee system are more diffuse when a consultant group rather than an individual consultant is used, but this diffusion is an asset in management of the transfer problem. The consultant group can more easily work with complex social systems because some division of labor is possible, and this arrangement is especially beneficial when transfer is necessary in order to introduce a consultant with skills different from those of the original consultant(s) to meet newly emerging problems in the consultee system.

Consultant-training programs that use an apprentice model may experience less difficulty with transfer, since the supervising consultant provides continuity in the consulting relationship. Mann (1973b) described an example of such an approach. Where the apprentice model is not used, maintenance of contact with the consultee system by the supervisor still provides the key to continuity in the relationship and introduction of new consultants to the system. Student consultants in the latter model can expect more exposure to entry-stage problems than those in the apprentice or group model, but this exposure is not necessarily undesirable from a training standpoint. The more critical issue is the benefit or lack of it that is attained by the consultee system in the light of regular consultant turnover. In extended consultation, the commitment of the consultant agency to maintaining the consulting relationship is critical to managing the transfer problem.

The question of transfer has implications for the planned duration of consulting programs and the selection of consultant training sites. Although consultation is conceived as a time-limited process under ideal conditions, those consultee systems that have a high degree of personnel turnover may profitably use consultation as a form of in-service training on a continuous basis. Such organizations provide desirable sites for training of students in consultation in a tradeoff relationship between the consultee and consultant-training organizations, as each is able to meet its training needs in this way. Stable organizations with little turnover, however, are likely to have more experienced personnel and may benefit more from time-limited, program- or system-focused consultation. This type of consultation does not preclude training, but the consultee system will not provide a continuous-training site in which the problem of consultant transfer needs to be anticipated. Time-limited consultation necessarily involves facing the issue of termination, a topic to be addressed next.

TERMINATION

Compared with the literature on the entry problem, the literature on termination in consultation is quite limited. Obviously it is easier to end a consultation, one way or another, than it is to begin one. Yet this fact should not obscure the importance of the termination process in achieving the goals of consultation. In a sense, the problem-solving nature of consultation requires that it focus on an end point as well as on processes, but often the desired end point is continuation of processes set in motion by the consultation as well as a more finite outcome.

In reality, the termination point of many consultations is defined by expiration of a preset period of time, such as the end of a demonstration period or expiration of grant funds. These predetermined points have no theoretical basis. From a theoretical standpoint, consultation relationships should reach a termination stage through mutual agreement between consultant and consultees that a satisfactory degree of progress toward goals has been achieved and that further progress depends upon increasingly independent action by the consultee system. This point may be determined by reference to evaluative data or by discussion of observations of consultees, or both. In any case, it is desirable that a decision to enter a termination stage be made through mutual agreement.

Management of the termination process varies with consultation methods. Caplan (1970, pp. 292-293), described a rather abrupt ending once his task has been completed, emphasizing his posture that the consultee system is then free to accept or reject the results of his work. He suggested subsequent follow-up to assess the effectiveness of the consultation. Schein (1969) spoke of termination as a process of disengagement, with the consultant gradually reducing involvement with the consultee system, but leaving the door open to subsequent brief reentry should the consultee system so desire. During the termination stage, the consultant reverts to a role that is similar to the one assumed during the familiarization process, observing consultee-system processes and serving as a sounding board against which the consultee system can test out ideas. Schein believed that gradual disengagement rather than a complete cessation of involvement affords an opportunity to test out the diagnostic hypothesis that the consultee system is ready for termination, a diagnosis that may not be correct. Maintenance of the possibility of reentry also provides an opportunity for follow-up similar to that suggested by Caplan.

The two primary tasks of termination, then, are mutual assessment of consultation effectiveness and management of residual dependencies on the consultant. As in psychotherapy, problems with dependency, or even with organizational stagnation during the consultation process, may be managed by strategic use of reduced consultant involvement without complete termination. Gradual withdrawal of the consultant may create a social vacuum that increases the forces within the organization to take over the functions formerly provided by the consultant, a development that may not occur in the consultant's presence. At other times, setting an ending date may force attention on the incompleted tasks that must be addressed prior to termination.

From a theoretical standpoint, both transfer and termination are special cases of the principal of succession in Kelly's adaptation (1968) of ecological concepts to psychological intervention. The succession principle underscores the evolutionary nature of human life and the recognition that, as one set of problems are resolved, new ones emerge. Following this principle, the consultant seeks to promote self-sufficiency of the organization and to avoid making the consultant function as an indispensable part of the consultee system. The alert consultant also recognizes that his or her particular relationship to the consultee system may be interrupted for any number of unforeseen circumstances, and gives some thought to the question of succession from the beginning of the relationship.

The question of termination usually implies a greater self-sufficiency on the part of the consultee system to meet those problems that led to initiation of the consultation relationship. The succession principle draws attention to the possible need to initiate a planned withdrawal or reduction in consultative contacts. It is, of course, possible to maintain a consultation relationship with only occasional contact to maintain or reaffirm the gains that have been made. In other circumstances, a transition in functions, rather than termination, may be indicated. As mentioned earlier, in systems with a high rate of personnel turnover, consultation may be used as a kind of in-service training, or other forms of in-service training may be implemented using the consultant to assist in program development and occasional training. For other consultee systems, evolutionary changes either within the system or outside of it may create needs for other kinds of consultation, in which case the entire process of problem definition and negotiation would be reopened. These processes are similar to those described in connection with the transfer of consultants discussed earlier.

An example of these processes can be provided from the author's own experience. This consultation was a 2-year, time-limited demonstration project on consultation and training with a police department (Mann, 1973b). At the end of the project, the author left the area to accept another position. The issue of succession was discussed with members of the consultee system, and arrangements were made for one of the graduate students who had worked on the project to continue the relationship. Since that time, a succession of consultants have been employed to meet a variety of emergent needs. At the time of this writing, this relationship has evolved to the point that the department has hired two full-time psychologists to provide consultation, training, and personal counseling for personnel in service. This transition has involved a greatly increased set of psychological functions, but, importantly, these functions have been made a part of the system itself, rather than continuing to rely on outside consultants. Other departments have adapted to their continuing need for such services by training police officers in providing these functions, although they often still rely on outside consultants to a degree. It seems likely that consultants operating out of a mental health setting will more often than not maintain some contact with consultee systems, at least in a liaison role around coordinating referrals, and may continue to provide occasional consultation and training.

As with other transition points in consultation, these are tasks that require sound judgment on the part of the consultant and openness and mutuality of communication with the consultee system. Assessment of the achievements of the consultation can be aided by making reference to the consultation contract. Understanding needs to be reached about collection and subsequent use of any further evaluative data. Any plans on the part of the consultant to publish information about the consultation should be discussed with the consultee system so that its rights to review any such material can be clarified. Similarly, an understanding should be reached concerning any future contact between consultant and consultee system, whether for follow-up or possible reentry.

In the final analysis, the effectiveness of the termination stage will depend on the accuracy of the diagnosis that the consultee system is ready for termination. In this regard, the gradual disengagement recommended by Schein would seem to have distinct advantages. As with the other transition points discussed here, viewing termination as a process provides an opportunity to use this stage to reinforce the gains achieved by the preceding consultation work.

NOTES

1. Mann. P. A. *Ethical issues for psychologists in the law enforcement system.* Paper presented to workshop of the Task Force on the Role of Psychology in the Criminal Justice System, Board of Social and Ethical Responsibility, American Psychological Association, Berkeley, Calif., February 1977.

2. Monahan, J. *Report of the Task Force on the Role of Psychology in the Criminal Justice System.* Board of Social and Ethical Responsibility, American Psychological Association, Washington, D.C., 1978.

3. Benjamin, C. M. *Consultee receptivity to consultation as a function of crisis.* Unpublished doctoral dissertation, University of Texas, Austin, 1967.
4. Burke, M. *The institution of the consultation process within a university context.* Unpublished doctoral dissertation, University of Texas, Austin, 1970.
5. Mann, P. A. A model for psychological consultation and training in a campus setting. Paper presented at American Personnel and Guidance Association meeting, Cleveland, 1974.

REFERENCES

Bennis, W. G. *Changing organizations.* New York: McGraw-Hill, 1966.

Caplan, G. *The theory and practice of mental health consultation.* New York: Basic Books, 1970.

Cherniss, C. Pre-entry issues in consultation. *American Journal of Community Psychology,* 1976, *4,* 13-24.

Glidewell, J. The entry problem in consultation. *Journal of Social Issues,* 1959, *15*(2), 51-59.

Heller, K., & Monahan, J. *Psychology and community change.* Homewood, Ill.: Dorsey Press, 1977.

Hirshman, R. Utilization of mental health consultation and self-perceptions of intraorganizational importance and influence. *Journal of Consulting and Clinical Psychology,* 1974, *42,* 916.

Jarvis, P. E., & Nelson, S. Familiarization: A vital step in mental health consultation. *Community Mental Health Journal,* 1967, *3,* 343-348.

Katz, D., & Kahn, R. L. *The social psychology of organizations.* New York: Wiley, 1966.

Kelly, J. G. Towards an ecological conception of preventive interventions. In J. W. Carter (Ed.), *Research contributions from psychology to community mental health.* New York: Behavioral Publications, 1968.

Levine, M. Some postulates of practice in community psychology and their implications for training. In I. Iscoe & C. D. Spielberger (Eds.), *Community psychology: Perspectives in training and research.* New York: Appleton-Century-Crofts, 1970.

Lewin, K. *Field theory in social science.* New York: Harper and Row, 1951.

Lippitt, R. Dimensions of the consultant's job. *Journal of Social Issues,* 1959, *15*(2), 5-12.

Mann, P. A. Accessibility and organizational power in the entry phase of mental health consultation. *Journal of Consulting and Clinical Psychology,* 1972, *38,* 215-218.

_____. Student consultants: Evaluations by consultees. *American Journal of Community Psychology,* 1973a, *1,* 182-193.

_____. *Psychological consultation with a police department.* Springfield, Ill.: Charles C. Thomas, 1973b.

118   THE MENTAL HEALTH CONSULTATION FIELD

———— & Iscoe, I. Mass behavior and community organization: Reflections on a peaceful demonstration. *American Psychologist,* 1971, *26,* 108-113.

Sarason, S. B., Levine, M., Goldenberg, I. I., Cherlin, D. L., & Bennett, E. M. *Psychology in community settings: Clinical, educational, vocational, social aspects.* New York: Wiley, 1966.

Schein, E. H. *Process consultation: Its role in organization development.* Reading, Mass.: Addison-Wesley, 1969.

Sofer, C. *The organization from within.* Chicago: Quadrangle Books, 1961.

Chapter 8

ACCOUNTABILITY AND ECONOMICS IN CONSULTATION

Milton F. Shore, Ph.D.
Fortune V. Mannino, Ph.D.

Changes in the mental health field with rising involvement of government (at all levels) in service delivery, competing priorities for tax revenues, more consumer input in service planning, greater focus on prevention, all coupled with national economic difficulties have led to great concern with fiscal issues, such as the sources of funds (financing) and the use of funds (accountability). Unlike in business and industry, where there has long been a concern with defining and measuring success, cost-containment and management-by-objectives, professional human services have been considered a societal good and such issues have gone relatively unquestioned in deference to the education and wisdom of the professional. No longer is this so, as professionals along with others have been challenged to prove through documentation that their services are worthwhile. In the past, society had given professionals certain rights because of their commitment to high-quality service. Fiscal matters were considered secondary to the provision of high-quality care. Today, the professional, like the business manager, has an obligation to relate service costs to quality of care. Just because a particular service costs more does not mean that the quality of that service is necessarily better. Professionals must ask, ''What are the most efficient, most effective, and least expensive ways of delivering a high-quality service in the short and the long run?

Nowhere are the issues of financing and accountability of mental health services more complex and difficult than when they are applied to consultation services. Questions can be asked: Of what value are indirect services? What evidence do we need to show that prevention is effective?

How can mental health consultation be most efficiently financed? How does one record statistics and keep records of such a difficult area?

This chapter will present some of the problems and issues of financing and accountability in mental health consultation. In contrast to many other aspects of mental health service delivery that have a longer tradition, the relatively new field of mental health consultation has not addressed many of these concerns. This chapter, therefore, is one of the first attempts to present for consideration the issues in accountability and financing. It focuses around what currently exists, not what should be. As the field grows and matures, we should be able to ask, "How should mental health resources (staff and funds) be best distributed to have the greatest impact on those in need?"

THE VALUE OF CONSULTATION

The potential value of mental health consultation lies not in just effecting personal change in a consultee, but in the fact that important changes in the social environment can be accomplished with the use of limited mental health personnel. Mental health consultation does not deal with individual patients; it does not base its work on psychopathology; it does not set as a goal providing corrective emotional experiences for those who have suffered a lack of social-psychological nourishment. It does not shy away from such problems, but approaches them on a different plane—that of the environment or the social context in which they occur.

From a conceptual viewpoint, the environment—an organization, community, society, or any of its subparts—is looked upon as consisting of forces and resources that can retard or interfere with social functioning as well as enhance and facilitate (Caplan & Grunebaum, 1972). The goal of mental health consultation is to improve the relationship between individuals and their social context by changing the balance of forces in the direction of facilitating and enhancing growth. Consultation accomplishes such change through the spread-of-effect phenomenon. Operationally this means that change in the behavior of a consultee, such as a teacher, will spread to others in the consultee's social environment through the consultee's interactions and interrelationships. Theoretically, bringing about personal change in a teacher can have an effect on the students in that teacher's classroom. Or, effecting change in a principal can have an impact on the mental health of the entire school. In this fashion the consultee becomes a mediator for further change and thus serves as a change agent in his or her own right.

Fortunately the preceding example is no longer based just on theory. Studies reporting on the outcome of consultation are increasing in both quantity and quality. Furthermore, researchers are expanding their criteria of change to include measurements of the social environment and the clientele as well as of the consultee. Out of 21 studies reported in the literature that examined change on the level of the clientele or social setting or some combination of the consultee, the social setting, and the clientele (all of which met minimum scientific standards including controls and testing hypotheses), 8 studies, or 38.1 percent, showed significant positive change as predicted and 9 others showed significant change in part. In total, 81.0 percent of the studies showed change in whole or in part. These findings are not as strong as one might hope for, but considering the tremendous complexities involved in conducting such research, they are certainly a sound beginning in establishing a base of data attesting to the validity of consultation as a method of community mental health practice and to the spread-of-effect phenomenon that it encompasses. These findings speak also to the economic advantages of consultation. By effecting change in the quantity of maladaptive behavior and/or improving the mental health elements of the social context in which behavior occurs with minimal professional staff, the intervention methodologies involved are inherently cost-effective, although specific data on cost have yet to come in.

It is for these reasons that consultation has grown as a viable, independent field autonomous from other mental health areas. It is becoming clear that consultation should not be linked indiscriminately with other services, but should set its own priorities, assess its own values, and operate as a separate service entity.

FINANCING CONSULTATION SERVICES

Despite the many advantages of mental health consultation activities, consultation is still the most difficult of all the mental health services to support financially, with less funding available than for any of the other mental health services. Mental health consultation takes up minimal amounts of staff and time in mental health agencies; recent estimates show consultation and education services taking 5 percent of the time in community mental health centers (Goldstein, 1977a).

The comprehensive concept that formed the basis of the Community Mental Health Centers Act of 1963 (Public Law 88-164) included a commitment to all aspects of mental health in the community. Included were indirect services, such as mental health consultation and education, as well as direct treatment services, such as inpatient and outpatient care. Because of the broad conception of mental health within a community context and the commitment to more than the treatment model, consultation and education were included as one of the five essential services in the original 1963 act. Yet development of community mental health centers (CMHCs) made no provision for how money was to be used and what balance there should be of direct and indirect services. Thus what happened over the 8-year decreased funding period set for centers was that less and less money was being used for consultation and education. Goldstein (1977a) presented data showing a steady increase in funding for indirect services until the eighth and final year of federal funding, at which point there was a marked decrease. A recent study by Abt Associates (Naierman, Haskins, Robinson, Zook, & Wilson, 1978) also indicate that the seed money approach was successful in initiating community mental health programs but that it did not guarantee that community mental health centers would continue to function in their original form after federal grants had been terminated.

Community mental health centers often changed their original form because providers of alternative funds had their own program priorities, which often differed from those of federal programs. One of these priorities, was a decline in indirect services and emphasis in areas such as partial hospitalization, emergency services, and inpatient services. Naierman et al. noted that satelite clinics, outreach services, and consultation-education services were the first areas for which funding was cut when the community mental health centers met with financial difficulty in their last year of federal support. The Abt study therefore recommended that seed money be followed by maintenance money to be used as leverage for negotiation for other funds.

A number of amendments to the Community Mental Health Centers Act since 1963 have had major significance for the funding of mental health consultation programs. In 1970, Public Law 91-211 expanded the staffing grants to permit further development of consultation and education services in all community mental health programs. Awareness of the difficulties consultation and education programs had in generating income led to the recommendation that staff be encouraged and supported in developing such programs. But again, no major fiscal policy changes took place.

It was in 1975 that a major thrust occurred with the passage of Public Law 94-63. The 1975 amendments recognized that consultation was funded by taking funds from other programs. Therefore funding of consultation and education programs as independent services was legislated and implemented using a highly complicated formula. This was the first time that funds were delegated separately to consultation services. In addition, the funding was not time limited. Consultation and education services were clearly defined in the legislation as being appropriate for a wide range of individuals and entities involved with mental health services, including health professionals, schools, courts, state and local law enforcement and correctional agencies, members of the clergy, public welfare agencies, health delivery systems, and other appropriate entities.

Public Law 94-63 also defined consultation and education services in terms of recipients and substantive areas. Differing from direct clinical service, consultation and education were to (1) develop effective mental health programs in the CMHC catchment area, (2) promote coordination of provision of mental health services among various entities serving the center's catchment area, (3) increase awareness of the residents of the center's catchment area of the nature of mental health problems and the types of mental health services available, and (4) promote prevention of rape and proper treatment of rape victims. The law provided consultation and education grants for programs that had never participated in the original community mental health center program as well as to centers that had completed their 8 years of support. In certain instances, centers currently receiving staffing operation grants were eligible for additional funds. Responsibility for the consultation and education program had to be shared by the governing body, a professional advisory board, and the center director, although day-to-day operational responsibility could be vested in a separate administrative unit coordinating consultation and education services.

In 1976, 55 new consultation and education grants averaging $77,900 each and totaling $3.9 million were awarded. Forty-one grants totaling some $3½ million were approved but could not be funded. In 1977, $3.6 million in grants was awarded (*Community Mental Health Center News,* January 1978). Yet, although these new consultation and education grants were helpful, the money allocated fell far short of being able to fund all the service programs approved and covered only a small proportion of the total number of community mental health centers. Thus funding continued to be a major problem for consultation and education services.

Slow Growth of Consultation Services

There are a number of reasons why mental health consultation services continued to have financial problems. Often consultation has as its goal prevention of mental illness. Despite the rhetoric, there has been generally very little commitment nationally to prevention of mental illness and promotion of mental health. The illness model, which historically formed the basis of the mental health movement, remains paramount, despite a growing interest in a health model. Treating mental illness is seen as top-priority. Of course, consultation that is educationally based may be focused more on alleviation of a specific problem than on prevention of the next problem. Certainly there are prevention strategies other than consultation.

A second factor slowing the funding of consultation is the lack of clarity in the field itself. Although consultation has been viewed as an indirect service, there are very few training programs and a very limited number of skilled practitioners in the area. As yet, standards have not been set for training, and clarification of what is needed to carry out a consultation and education service of first quality has not been delineated.

A third area limiting fiscal growth has been the problems involved in conducting outcome research on mental health consultation. The difficulties inherent in doing research on indirect services are greater than those present in doing research on direct services. Major conceptual, methodological, and measurement issues still remain (Mannino & Shore, 1975).

A fourth factor slowing progress is budget constraints. When budgets become tight, one has to make choices. The fiscal choices made are often in terms of more traditional and less risky ways of working. Schools, for example, are a major source of consultation services. Currently under a budget crunch, many schools have decided to pull back their sources of funding and to either develop direct services within their own school systems, reduce their mental health services, put more money into the education that is seen as their primary task, or change the ways their own personnel work, rather than hire consultants from outside the system.

A fifth area related to difficulties in funding consultation services is that the potential recipient of consultation, that is, the person who is desirous of and acknowledges the need for such services, may not be the same person who pays for it. This may mean convincing an administrator with little or no understanding of consultation that the service can benefit the organization.

One further reason for difficulty in funding consultation and education is insurance. Insurance companies reimburse for direct, rather than indirect, services and rarely reimburse for preventive services. Services have grown in proportion to the availability of third-party payments; that is, development follows the easy availability of funds.

Sources of Funding for Consultation Programs

Given these constraints, what are some current sources of funding for consultation services?

1. The major source of funding for consultation services has been government at federal, state, county, or local levels. Over the years, there

has been greater recognition that public funds should be appropriated for consultation as well as treatment services.

2. Community mental health centers have become more and more involved in billing for third-party payments. In case consultation, where contracts are written for diagnostic types of services employing a classical medical consultative model, reimbursement from third-party payers is straightforward, albeit not always granted. Gaining reimbursement for non-case-oriented consultation, however, has been difficult, if not impossible.

3. A fee-for-service model has been used in some community mental health centers. In Pennsylvania, for example, agencies pay for courses given to staff (*ADAMHA News,* November 9, 1977). With the current budget problems in agencies, the opportunity to contract with outside agencies for in-service training and consultation becomes less available. If ways can be found for staff members to obtain continuing education credits or other rewards for work with a consultant, then, perhaps, agencies might be more willing to subsidize consultant activities. Nevertheless, the fee-for-service model has great potential for increasing volume and maintaining consistency and certainly needs to be explored further.[1]

4. Foundation grants, although available, have been minimal and are unpredictable. Many foundations are willing to initiate some activities and give seed money, but are not willing to fund for extended periods of time. Similarly, personal gifts are also unpredictable. A strategy used with success by some agencies has been for the consultant to assist the community agency in applying for grant or contract funds.

There seems no doubt that there is a need for creative thought to be given to developing new strategies for funding consultation programs. A number of current trends offer some new opportunities for more funding and bode well for the future:

1. The President's Commission on Mental Health stressed the area of prevention services, suggesting that ultimately 10 percent of the budget of the National Institute of Mental Health be used for prevention (*Report to the President,* 1978). How prevention will be defined and how mental health consultation will be included in the prevention initiative are issues that remain to be explored.

2. The current concern with continuing education offers many opportunities for training. Perhaps continuing education credits could be given to consultees since consultation is a learning experience.

3. Prepaid medical groups, such as health maintenance organizations (HMOs), have been encouraged to cut medical costs. To reduce costs, these plans stress early identification and prevention. Since consultation is potentially an efficient and economical way of delivering services consistent with those goals, many of these HMOs may undertake more consultation programming.

4. Capitation funding, where funds for services, especially public funds, will be distributed on the basis of catchment area population, may foster more consultation because of the ceiling on population income. Such a ceiling forces employment of more efficient ways of using financial resources.

5. A major issue is how indirect services may be funded in a national health insurance program. How will indirect services be defined in such a program? Should a national health insurance program have provisions for innovative health promotion activities, or will there be two types of funding: a national health insurance program for direct services and federal grants and contracts available for indirect services, as suggested by Borus (1978)?

6. If implemented, one of the specific recommendations of the President's Commission on Mental Health may profoundly affect funding of mental health consultation programs. The Task Panel on Community Supports urged that Title XX legislation be amended to allow such community institutions and organizations as schools, religious organizations, and voluntary associations to receive funds for mental health consultation and education services (*Task Panel Reports*, 1978).

In summary, the funding of mental health consultation has been exceedingly difficult for theoretical, political, professional, and practical reasons. Current concerns with costs, however, may lead to more efficient use of resources as we develop prevention programs and evaluate the various funding strategies. Indeed, mental health consultation should profit from such a reorganization, redistribution, and rethinking of the mental health field and its relationship to personal and social problems.

ACCOUNTABILITY AND CONSULTATION

As it becomes increasingly necessary to seek out new sources of financial support for consultation programming, it becomes even more important to be able to show that resources are being used in an accountable manner. The need for accountability in professional practice is not new to professionals in the human service field. The recent urgency seems to stem from the increased public expenditures, particularly by the federal government, in mental health service delivery, or as one author put it, "the shift from the domain of families, neighborhood, and employers to the public sector" (Stretch, 1978, p. 323). This increase in federal expenditures has resulted in the need for governmental agencies (spurred on by investigations by such private groups as Ralph Nader's and such official auditing agencies as the General Accounting Office) to give greater attention to issues of accountability and evaluation. This, in turn, has led to including accountability in such federal legislation as Public Law 94-63 and extending concern beyond procedural issues to substantive regulation of programs (Goldstein, 1977b).

Significance for Consultation

This trend toward standards and accountability is common to all components of community mental health (and to all human service efforts in general), but mental health consultation programs are especially vulnerable. Mental health consultation has been the primary vehicle for extending services into the community and for coordinating mental health services with other community health and social service programs. Often such activities have necessitated development of creative programs to reach particularly difficult high-risk groups and other populations with special needs and problems. Such efforts are encouraged when resources are plentiful, but they are extremely vulnerable when the trend is toward greater efficiency, efficacy, and accountability. Added to these problems are the inherent difficulties in establishing criteria and standards for evaluation of consultation services. As already mentioned, there are no generally acceptable standards for the practice of consultation. Thus in many ways the current emphasis on accountability has greater significance for the survival of consultation than for other components of care, particularly the more traditional, direct services.

Consultation as a field also requires a conceptual reorientation and changes in the way of viewing how services are delivered. As compared with accountability in direct services, accountability in indirect services must deal also with the issue of for whom consultants are working. Are they accountable to the agency, the consultee, and/or the client? In this regard, what new issues of confidentiality arise? Is each contact a "case": Is the relationship with the consultee privileged? What are the issues when various parts of the system are in conflict and the consultant sees that the clients are affected (Fanibanda, 1976; Haylett, 1969)?

Internal and External Accountability

One of the main complaints made by the General Accounting Office (the primary auditing body of the Congress of the United States), in its investigation of the community mental health centers programs, was that the centers' evaluation efforts were of little value because the amount of time taken delayed results until after program decisions were made and/or that the quality of results was of little value in the decision-making process (General Accounting Office, 1974). In other words, there was no internal accountability, no way for the centers to show themselves that their programs were operating in an effective and efficient manner. A similar criticism was made by the Nader group. Indeed, their main criterion used to judge the success or failure of an evaluation program was whether the program collected information that was useful in policy decision making (Chu & Trotter, 1974). Internal accountability therefore relates to information the program administrator must have. To quote Chapman:

> If the manager of a mental health organization doesn't know whether expectations of service are being met, he can't tell what to do about existing programs. If he doesn't know what clientele is being served and can't compare it with the community's total needs, he does not know what services he should develop. If he doesn't know what services are being delivered, he can't determine their effectiveness. If he doesn't know the cost of existing services, he can't estimate the cost of different services and make informed judgments about efficient allocation of resources. (Chapman, 1976, p. 8)

This then, is the core of internal accountability: the process of program decision making based on data relevant to current program characteristics and community needs.

When questions similar to the preceding ones are asked by an external agency, such as the federal government, external accountability comes into play. As already noted, the frequency of external agencies' asking such questions about program operations has increased manyfold over the past decade. As consultation programs seek new funding sources, external demands for evidence of accountability can also be expected to increase. Fortunately there is considerable overlap in the kinds of information needed for internal and external accountability, so that a program with an information system capable of assuring one will also go a long way toward assuring the other (Sorenson & Grove, 1978).

Information Systems

Generally speaking, some information is gathered by all mental health agencies, but usually on a catch-as-catch-can basis rather than routinely and systematically. Unfortunately this leads to rather loose programming, that is, programming based on special interests and/or staff impressions or prejudices and goals that are arbitrary and idiosyncratically determined, with only (at best) minimal responsiveness to community needs and problems. Moreover, no structure is provided for future program development and for program evaluation. What is called for, particularly in the area of consultation, is a data-based, rational program with planning dynamically linked to the ongoing life of the community, its problems, needs, and systems of support, both formal and informal, with the desired results (outcome) stated clearly and explicitly in measurable terms. Information systems can aid development of this process immensely when the information is used as part of program decision making.

The key to information systems is continuous collection of the kinds of data that can have a meaningful influence on program planning and operations. Two major questions are: What kinds of information can serve as a continuous source of program guidance? What mechanisms are available for collecting it?

The kinds of information needed can best be described in terms of five major assessment areas: community needs and problems, program effort, recipient groups, program costs, and program progress and outcome. These are shown in Table 8-1 along with the primary type of information required in each area. As can be seen, there are two levels of information: (1) information concerned with characteristics of the community or environment and (2) information concerned with program characteristics.

Mechanisms for collecting information about the community are referred to as *Community Monitoring Systems* or *Community Information Systems,* and mechanisms for collecting information about program characteristics are called *Management Information Systems.* Both are important. Also necessary is a way to link the two systems of information so that program efforts can be related to community needs. One way of accomplishing such a linkage is by having certain basic elements of information, such as census tract identification, from both systems correspond (Broskowski, 1977).

Information systems in the area of direct services have been used for some time, and considerable progress has been made. Only recently, however, have such systems been developed for collecting information on consultation and indirect services (Cytrynbaum, 1974; Broskowski, Driscoll, & Schulberg, 1978; Flaherty, 1977; Ketterer & Bader, 1977; Hagedorn, Beck, Neubert, & Werlin, 1976; Chapman, 1976; and Mannino & MacLennan, 1978).

Community Information System

A Community Information System is essential for operating a community health program in general, but has special significance for planning and operating a consultation program. (Indeed, planning a consulta-

TABLE 1

Major Assessment Areas	Examples of Type of Information Needed
I. Assessment of Community Needs and Problems	High-risk population groups. Other population groups with special needs. Population groups with inadequate resources. Acute problems and crises.
II. Assessment of Effort	Number of staff providing consultation (by discipline, position and recipients). Types of consultation being provided (by discipline, position and recipients). Staff hours devoted to consultation (by discipline, position and recipients). Effort pattern (current vs. past years).
III. Assessment of Recipient Groups	Recipient agencies, their location and target groups (social and demographic characteristics of target groups). Pattern of recipient agencies compared with previous years.
IV. Assessment of Program Costs	Consultants by discipline, activity, location. Problem and method. Time involved (preparation, travel to and from location, actual consultation session, preparation of reports). Pattern of expenditures over time.
V. Assessment of Program Progress and Outcome	Progress notes showing specific goals and accomplishments. Information for peer review re: adequacy of progress. Process and outcome measures, e.g., Satisfaction Questionnaires, Expectation Measures, Goal Achievement Scales.

tion program without relevant information about the community is akin to a psychotherapist's planning a treatment program for a patient he or she knows nothing about.) This need for an information system is due to the community nature of consultation as a method of intervention, its orientation based on population groups, its liaison function, its special sensitivity to community needs and problems, and its role in developing new resources and reshaping community delivery systems.

One important source of community/environment information is the Mental Health Demographic Profile System (MHDPS) developed by the National Institute of Mental Health, now available for each community mental health catchment area in the country and adaptable as well to other planning areas. This system is able to provide a picture of the characteristics of dominant and subdominant population groups in a census tract of a catchment area. Based on census materials, the most objective and complete set of national data available, it includes socioeconomic status, ethnic composition, household composition and family structure, lifestyles, and housing and community instability and operates on the assumption that population characteristics are associated with social behavior. It permits rough approximation of high-risk groups in a particular social area in terms of need for mental health and other types of social services and is able to point to specific populations with special needs, such as the elderly, families in poverty, or widowed females (Rosen, Lawrence, Goldsmith, Windle, & Shambaugh, 1975). It therefore presents a large picture of the community analogous to an aerial view, while at the same time pointing to areas that need closer examination. It may show that, for example, a particular census tract contains a large population of elderly people, but it does not show what kinds of supports, both formal and informal, are available or what the service gaps are between needs and resources. Hence it screens an area and provides cues as to where finer focusing is required. In another tract containing mostly very young children and their families, the need is to focus on the supports available to this population group to determine the most strategic contacts for consultation—perhaps a day care program, nursery schools, health centers, kindergartens, or pediatricians. Whatever the final program choices may be, the important point is being able to differentiate programs in accordance with the data to ensure their relevance to community realities (Gabbay & Windle, 1975).

To complement the rather global picture of the community provided by the census data, there is a need for a mechanism that allows closer scrutiny of specific parts of the community, that is, one that systematically collects naturalistic, descriptive data so as to provide a regularly updated information source for the consultation program. In the census tract with a

132 THE MENTAL HEALTH CONSULTATION FIELD

large population of elderly people, for example, much more information about this community subarea is needed to facilitate consultation program planning. One needs information about housing, shopping, health, transportation, recreation, churches, social services, adult education, informal helping networks. Also helpful is information regarding particular problems, social forces, and other factors impacting on persons living in this area. In brief, one needs as complete a picture as possible to assist in a comprehensive assessment of the area, in terms of both needs and resources. Only then can one hope to plan and develop a rational consultation program grounded in the realities of the community.

These kinds of naturalistic, descriptive data can be of considerable help to a consultation program in other ways, for instance, in having to make quick assessments of areas in which a community crisis or disaster has occurred, when time becomes a significant factor in program planning; as a resource for consultants on how particular neighborhoods or other parts of the community went about solving certain problems, such as vandalism or child care for working parents; to identify leaders from particular parts of the community for consideration as candidates for the agency's board, committees, coordinating planning bodies; to provide clues as to the possible reactions of different community areas to establishment of such facilities as a halfway house for juvenile offenders or a cooperative housing program for returning mental patients. No doubt there are many additional ways this information can be used that have not been mentioned.

One mechanism for collecting this type of naturalistic information based on the *Community File System* developed at the Mental Health Study Center, was described in a monograph by Mannino and MacLennan (1978). Establishing a Community File System takes staff effort and organizational ability, but the information is readily available to any agency. A Community File System is compiled mainly by identifying and locating the sources of available community information, arranging for its regular collection, and then processing and storing it so that it is readily available to the consultation staff. A well-established Community File System would contain formal documents and reports from all the agencies, organizations, civic associations, churches, schools, clubs, and hospitals located in the community served. It would contain news items from bulletins, newsletters, local newspapers, clubs, and other relevant sources. In addition, it would contain invaluable anecdotal material reported by staff in their travels around the community and in attendance at Parent-Teacher Association functions, agency open houses, and meetings of various kinds. The only limitation placed on the information collected is that placed on the consultation staff itself. Indeed, the Community File

System may be the one example of a situation in which it is permissible to collect data for some (currently unknown) future use with little fear that the data may never be used.

Program Information System

The second system of information, sometimes referred to as a Management Information System, is concerned with the collection of information about program characteristics. Basically there are two major areas of program information. The first is the area of how agency resources are used (effort); the second is the area of who are the recipients of the consultation effort. Often mentioned as a third area is expenses (Broskowski et al., 1978).

The Program Information System is concerned with the internal operations of an agency's consultation program. It asks broadly what the agency is doing by way of its consultation program to achieve its goals. In greater detail, it asks who is doing what, when, how, where, for whom, how long it has taken, and how much it costs. This is basically the same information required for the assessments shown in the second through fifth areas in Table 8-1.

The second and third areas in Table 8-1 deal specifically with the amounts and types of consultation provided and the number and types of recipients of the consultation. Hence they characterize the amount of effort expended, the recipients of the effort, and the characteristics of the client population served by the recipient group. When this information is related to the information collected about community needs (area 1), it is possible to make an assessment of the effectiveness of the consultation program in addressing community needs, an important factor in accountability. The Program Information System also furnishes the basis of information needed for planning programs and determining future program directions.

Related to the information in regard to effort is the information required for assessing costs. In the field of consultation, as in other areas of health care, costs of activities are closely related to effort expended by discipline and position, location of the activity, method of intervention, and amount of overall time required. To a large extent, costs may be differentiated along these variables, allowing programmers to establish units of cost for a consultation program package. In this manner, the costs of different kinds of consultation activities as well as the costs of consultation in relation to other helping modes may be compared (Broskowski, 1977).

Another important area related to accountability is program outcome. Generally outcome studies are a step beyond what can be accomplished with data collected through information systems, requiring greater scientific rigor, use of controls, and greater expense. Service programs should not be expected to carry out scientifically designed research to demonstrate the effectiveness of the various consultation service interventions used. This task is better left to research-oriented centers equipped with the necessary resources and expertise to conduct high-quality service delivery research (Hargreaves & Attkisson, 1978). Ideally such research in the area of consultation should be guided by a long-range research agenda established by a national-level advisory group made up of leaders in the field. Provisions could be made for regular reporting to service facilities whenever there is evidence to demonstrate the effectiveness (or ineffectiveness) of particular consultation intervention strategies.

This does not mean that agencies should not routinely collect hard data related to program progress and outcome designed to enhance the quality of their services. In the area of consultation, it is possible to collect information via progress reporting, as shown in area 5 of Table 8-1, that would allow an assessment of the adequacy of the progression of a consultation activity from inception to termination. In addition, some form of goal achievement could be incorporated as part of a progress report. If goals are stated in concrete and measurable terms, they may deal with either process variables, such as number of consultation sessions and number of participants, or with outcome variables, such as specific changes in communication or reduction in the number of problem children in a classroom. Kiresuk and Sherman (1968) developed the Goal Attainment Scale (GAS). Looking at consultation, the GAS might be set up as a scale on improving communication in an agency, varying from the least favorable outcome expected (e.g., "no change in communication") to the most favorable outcome expected (e.g., "open discussions and shared planning and decision making established"). A system for assigning weights and scoring the GAS was also developed by Kiresuk, Hagedorn et al., (1976).

When appropriate and relevant information regarding process and outcome is included routinely in progress recording, the records can be used as a system of review to monitor quality and assure accountability. Such a review could be done by peers, a formally constituted review committee, a supervisor, or perhaps members working as a team. In any event, the review process should be made an integral part of the assessment procedure. An excellent example of one approach toward building in a system of review, at the Yale-New Haven Community Mental Health Center, was described by Cytrynbaum (1974).

Implementation

To date there are no tried-and-true methods for implementing a Program Information System for mental health consultation. Many mental health facilities are in the process of testing and refining recordkeeping systems, reporting forms, and monitoring procedures. Examples of these were included in recent publications by Chapman (1976), Cytrynbaum (1974), Hagedorn et al. (1976), MacLennan, Montgomery, and Stern (1970), Montague and Taylor (1971), Beigel and Levenson (1978), and Mannino and MacLennan (1978). Although these can be used as guides for agencies struggling with development of information systems, specifics pertaining to what information to collect, how to collect it, and whether it should be processed automatically or by some type of hand sort must be determined by the individual agency's needs and resources.

SUMMARY

Information systems should be regarded as a service of the agency. If designed well and used systematically, they can help to tighten agency structure, facilitate communication among staff and between staff and management, and ensure greater responsiveness to the needs of the community and increased collaboration with formal and informal supports in the community. Although it should not be regarded as a research activity, data collection can certainly be used for research purposes. There is no reason for those agencies having the necessary resources and expertise not to engage in research if able to do so. The two activities should not be confused, however. They serve different masters, are judged by different criteria, and perform different functions. Research activities can enhance an agency's functioning by complementing and supplementing the work of an information system. Research, for example, can add to a program through additional studies of outcome and process of different consultation methodologies. It can focus down in a narrow and in-depth way and produce findings complementary to the more global picture gained from information systems.

CONCLUDING COMMENTS

Financing and accountability are seen by many professionals as primarily management and operational issues that are of little interest to the practitioner or service provider. The need for dealing with such issues has often caught the practitioner unawares. As with the politics of mental health, ignoring the issues does not make them go away. Indeed, in this case the reverse is usually true; that is, the issues grow larger and more visible, solutions become increasingly technical and managerial, and as a result program control is placed in the hands of people who are neither knowledgeable about nor vested in the delivery of mental health services.

Rather than bemoan the need to become involved in the issues, it behooves the mental health professional to use this current concern to advance the consultation field. The emphasis on quality of care, performance standards, and effective and efficient services requires a more organized and rational practice stance by consultants. Goals and objectives must be clearly formulated and related to carefully identified problems, clearly delineated target groups, and relevant modes of intervention. The immediate effect of this process is more rigorous and administratively viable consultation programs. In the long run, however, the entire field stands to benefit: concepts get defined and refined, training becomes clearer and more focused, problems in evaluation (especially such difficult evaluations as evaluating prevention) become sharper, and the discipline becomes more precise and effective. Thus professional leadership in this area not only can serve to effect much needed alterations in the structure and organization of service programs, but also can make significant and meaningful contributions toward advancing consultation as a field practice.

NOTES

1. Ediger, E. M. Personal communication, July 1978.

REFERENCES

ADAMHA News, November 9, 1977, p. 4.

Beigel, A., & Levenson, A. I. Program evaluation on a shoestring budget. In C. C. Attkisson, W. A. Hargreaves, M. J. Horowitz, & J. E. Sorensen (Eds.), *Evaluation of human service programs*. New York: Academic Press, 1978.

Borus, J. F. Issues critical to the survival of community mental health. *American Journal of Psychiatry*, 1978, *135*(9), 1029-1035.

Broskowski, A. Management information systems for planning and evaluation in human services. In I. Davidoff, M. Guttentag, & J. Offut (Eds.), *Evaluating community mental health services* (DHEW Pub. [ADM] 77-465). Rockville, Md.: National Institute of Mental Health, 1977.

————, Driscoll, J., & Schulberg, H. A management information and planning system for indirect services. In C. C. Attkisson, W. A. Hargreaves, M. J. Horowitz, & J. E. Sorensen (Eds.), *Evaluation of human service programs*. New York: Academic Press 1978.

Caplan, G., & Grunebaum, H. Perspectives on primary prevention. In H. Gottesfeld (Ed.), *Critical issues of community mental health*. New York: Behavioral Publications, 1972.

Chapman, R. L. *The design of management information systems for mental health organizations: A primer* (NIMH, DHEW Pub. [ADM] 76-333). Washington, D.C.: U.S. Government Printing Office, 1976.

Chu, F. D., & Trotter, S. *The madness establishment: Ralph Nader's study group report on the national institute of mental health.* New York: Grossman, 1974.

Community Mental Health Centers News, 1978, *9*(5), 3-4.

Cytrynbaum, S. A model for criteria-oriented review of consultation activities. In D. C. Riedel, G. Tischler, & J. Myers (Eds.), *Patient care evaluation in mental health programs.* Cambridge, Mass.: Ballinger, 1974.

Fanibanda, D. K. Ethical issues of mental health consultation. *Professional Psychology,* 1976, *8*(4), 547-552.

Flaherty, E. W. *A process-and-goal oriented management information system for CMHC consultation activities.* Paper presented at the Annual Meeting of the National Council of Community Mental Health Centers, Atlanta, 1977.

Gabbay, M., & Windle, C. *Demographic data to improve services: A sample of mental health applications.* Rockville, Md.: National Institute of Mental Health, 1975.

General Accounting Office. *Need for more effective management of community mental health centers program* (No. B-164031 [5]). Washington, D.C.: 1974.

Goldstein, L. S. *CMHCs, P.L. 94-63, and the clinical challenge of consultation and education services.* Paper presented to the National Committee for Mental Health Education, Atlanta, March 1977(a).

————. *Government concerns in the care of the mentally ill.* Paper presented at the 130th Annual Meeting of the American Psychiatric Association, Toronto, 1977(b).

Hagedorn, H. J., Beck, K. J., Neubert, S. F., & Werlin, S. H. *A working manual of simple program evaluation techniques for community mental health centers* (DHEW Pub. [ADM] 76-404). Rockville, Md.: National Institute of Mental Health, 1976.

Hargreaves, W. A., & Attkisson, C. C. Evaluating program outcomes. In C. C. Attkisson, W. A. Hargreaves, M. J. Horowitz, & J. E. Sorensen (Eds.), *Evaluation of human service programs.* New York: Academic Press, 1978.

Haylett, C. H. Issues of indirect services. In H. R. Lamb, D. Heath, & J. F. Downing (Eds.), *Handbook of community mental health practice.* San Francisco: Jossey-Bass, 1969.

Ketterer, R. F., & Bader, B. C. *Issues in the development of consultation and education services in community mental health centers.* Ann Arbor, Mich.: Center for Human Services Research, 1977.

Kiresuk, T. J., & Sherman, R. E. Goal attainment scaling: A general method for evaluating comprehensive community mental health programs. *Community Mental Health Journal,* 1968, *4,* 443-453.

MacLennan B., Montgomery, S., & Stern, E. *The analysis and evaluation of the consultation component in a community mental health center* (Laboratory Paper 36). Adelphi, Md.: Mental Health Study Center, NIMH, 1970.

Mannino, F. V., & MacLennan, B. *Monitoring and evaluating mental health consultation and education services* (DHEW Pub. [ADM] 77-550). Rockville, Md.: National Institute of Mental Health, 1978.

———, & Shore, M. F. The effects of consultation. *American Journal of Community Psychology*, 1975, *(1)*, *1-21*.

Mental Health Study Center, NIMH. *Community Characteristics Classification System Operating Manual*. Adelphi, Md.: Author (no date).

Montague, E. K., & Taylor, E. N. *Preliminary handbook on procedures for evaluating mental health indirect service programs in schools.* Alexandria, Va.: Human Resources Research Organization, 1971.

Naierman, N., Haskins, B., Robinson, G., Zook, C., & Wilson, D. *Community mental health centers: A decade later.* Cambridge, Mass.: Abt Books, 1978.

Report to the president from the President's Commission on Mental Health, Vol. I. Washington, D.C.: U.S. Government Printing Office, 1978, pp. 51-54.

Rosen, B. M., Lawrence, L., Goldsmith, H., Windle, C., & Shambaugh, J. *Mental health demographic profile system description: Purpose, contents and sampler of uses* (DHEW Pub. [ADM] 76-263). Rockville, Md.: National Institute of Mental Health, 1975.

Sorensen, J. E., & Grove, H. D. Using cost-outcome and cost-effectiveness analyses for improved program management and accountability. In C. C. Attkisson, W. A. Hargreaves, M. J. Horowitz, & J. E. Sorensen (Eds.), *Evaluation of human service programs,* New York: Academic Press, 1978.

Stretch, J. J. Increasing accountability for human services administrators. *Social Casework,* June 1978, *59*, 323-335.

Task panel reports submitted to the President's Commission on Mental Health, Vol. II Appendix. Washington, D.C.: U.S. Government Printing Office, 1978, p. 146.

Chapter 9

ETHICAL ISSUES AND CRITERIA IN INTERVENTION DECISIONS

Ronald Lippitt, Ph.D.

As professional people-helpers—working with individuals or groups or organizations or communities—we want to make the wisest decisions we can about what help is needed and how to be helpful.

Some of the guidelines we use for making these decisions are tactical and strategic: criteria about timing, readiness, probable consequences, risks, motivation. Other guidelines are values that are reflected in our answers to such questions as ''Are we the right helper?'' ''Are we creating dependency or learning?'' ''Is the potential change desirable or undesirable?''

The challenges for all of us are

1. To clarify the values we hold about our people-helping decisions and actions

2. To develop skill in using these values as part of our intervention decisions and behavior

3. To learn how to collect the data we need from our interactions with clients so we can continue to check and revise our values and our applications of them

I think of some of the guiding values as core values that help define the total posture toward the people-helping role. Other values are much more concrete and specific, applying to the making of specific decisions in particular situations.

139

Many hundreds of consultants and trainers, since 1947, have become aware of and have been guided by the core value statements developed by Benne and summarized most recently in his chapter on "The conceptual and moral foundations of laboratory method" (Benne, Bradford, Gibb, & Lippitt, 1975).

Let me very briefly summarize these seven "methodological values" for people-helpers, because they serve as basic guidelines for deriving the specific values needed to help clarify intervention decisions of consultants:

1. The processes of giving help *should be experimental,* aimed at developing more adequate ways of thinking about values and of handling a partly unknown future. The provisional plans should include a commitment to continuing evaluation and revision in the light of feedback on the consequences of the experiments.

2. The processes of helping *should be two-way interaction and influence.* This is a brief value statement of MacGregor's observation that a consultant will be listened to and influential with a client to the degree that the client perceives himself as able to influence the consultant.

3. Appropriate interventions *must be oriented toward objectively confronting tasks and situations,* not toward maintaining or augmenting the prestige or status needs and systems of the client or the consultant. In other words, a criterion of a relevant contribution is to ignore such categories as "expert," "experienced," "very young," and "in charge."

4. Processes of helping *should include objectives and techniques for supporting a process of learning and of learning how to learn or relearn* on the part of all the clients who are involved. This implies that one of the criteria of effective consultation is the enlarged capacity of the client to learn how to cope with succeeding problem situations without the collaboration of the consultant.

5. Appropriate procedures of helping *include efforts to search for and make full use of available relevant information and experience.* This rejects the notion that the consultant is the major resource and accepts the idea that one of her or his responsibilities is being a link to other resources.

6. Appropriate helping *rejects the notion of individual adjustment and personal independence* as the major objective of the helping process. This value perspective is one of regarding all client units as parts of interdependent systems in which there is a voluntary assumption of responsibility to give and take and to grow and solve problems through mutual processes of growth and development.

7. Appropriate helping processes *must provide for procedures of self-evaluation, self-correction, and self-renewal* of both the consultant and the client. This includes the notion of openness to the revision of values and goals as well as of techniques and means.

I will try to indicate below how these core values about helping can provide some of the basic guidelines from which one can derive guidance in specific intervention situations.

SOME CRITICAL INTERVENTION DECISIONS

From work with many consultants on development of our competencies as consultants, I have selected the following intervention decision situations as critical and illustrative of many more where values and ethical criteria are important components of the decision. A fuller inventory of intervention decision issues can be found in "Intervention Decisions and Actions: Dilemmas, Strategies, and Learnings" in Lippitt and Lippitt (1978).

I have found it helpful to organize intervention decisions under six phases of the consultant process. One can use these six phases to cluster the illustrative intervention decisions described later.

Phase 1. Initial Contact and Entry

Whom is it appropriate to define as the client?

How appropriate is it to state a need and express an expectation of being able to help without having a great deal of diagnostic information?

How can I demonstrate expertness and establish credibility as a source of help without creating dependence and expectations that I will "solve the problem"?

How can I be reassuring without my actions being interpreted as implying that the problem can be easily and quickly solved?

Phase 2. Formulating a Contract; Establishing a Working Relationship

How can I appropriately emphasize to clients their responsibilities and commitments for doing work without frightening them into withdrawal?

How can I clarify my own level of time and commitment without creating mistrust and apprehension?

How can I develop the necessary time perspective about the working-through process without appearing to be promoting more work for myself?

How can I communicate a trust and respect for clients' resourcefulness without buying into their diagnosis of the problem?

Phase 3. Problem Identification and Diagnosis

How can I maintain my belief in needed fact finding in the face of restricted openness and accessibility of data? This is a frequent conflict of interest.

How do I balance my interest, competence, and sophisticated diagnostic fact finding skill and the need to have the clients involved in ownership of the data?

Phase 4. Goal Setting and Planning

To what degree or when should I share preferred goals that I may have for clients?

To what degree should I suggest what I perceive as appropriate orientation toward the future?

How far can I push my values about who needs to be involved in the goal-setting and planning process?

Should I have goals for change in clients which I do not share?

Phase 5. Converting Plans into Action

How can I deal with the issues of mandated assignments versus voluntary commitments to participate in the implementation?

How can I deal with my need and clients' pressure for me to use my experience to produce the action?

How do I deal with my belief that the actions they are planning are inappropriate or ill advised and potentially harmful to others or to themselves?

Phase 6. Contract Completion: Continuity and Support

How can I communicate my beliefs about clients' needs for continuing support without being perceived as self-serving?

How can I communicate my belief in the responsibility of the client for documentation and dissemination of learning and successes?

How can I deal with my values about disclosure and confidentiality in sharing my learning from this client with others who would profit by it?

This is just a sample of the great variety of decisions and evaluations that must be a continuous part of the consultant's decision-making repertoire. If we are to function effectively, we need to develop procedures and skills for verifying and using value criteria as a part of every intervention decision we make in attempting to provide help and support to clients.

SOME SAMPLES OF DECISION MAKING

Decision 1. Who Is My Client?

The Situation. The administrator of the center asks me to "help them resolve their conflict" about duplication of services to clients. "Them" is the community outreach unit, headed by a clinical psychologist, and the volunteer services team, headed by a social group worker.

The Decision Dilemma. Shall I regard the administrator as client and work out a helping contract with him, or shall I regard the two unit leaders or the two units as my clients?

Some Decision-Action Alternatives as I See Them

1. Accept the request as legitimate

2. Ask the administrator to involve the two units and get their acceptance of my helper role

3. Tell the administrator I will need to meet with the two unit heads and find out whether they can accept client relationship to me

4. Ask the adminstrator to convene the relevant parties to meet with me to explore readiness and possibility of taking client role with me

Value Criteria I Feel the Need to Consider and Use

1. The administrator has the right and responsibility to intervene to improve the quality of service rendered by his staff.

2. I do not believe it is ethical to try to influence the decisions and behavior of persons who have not accepted my right to try to help them.

3. I believe a large proportion of those who need help do not accept this need or feel able to ask for help, so "selling them on me" is appropriate.

4. The administrator probably is a crucial part of the system, to be worked with if a significant solution is to be found and maintained.

5. I think I am an appropriate resource for this type of problem.

6. Other criteria readers may discover as you review this and think about it further.

The Decisions and Actions of This Consultant

1. I told the administrator I was challenged by the problem and thought there was a good chance I could help.

2. But I could not agree to work on it unless we could get agreement from the unit heads and perhaps the units.

3. I agreed that the administrator might have difficulty getting non-coerced cooperation or avoiding setting up counterdependent resistance, so I suggested I should take some responsibility for "selling" my service, if he would sanction my making contact with the two unit heads.

4. I stated that if I could develop their readiness to work with me, I would expect a three-way meeting, including him, to arrive at a mutual agreement on my role, my time, their time, my access to their units, etc. "They" will be the client.

Some Value Principles Utilized

1. The working contract with the client should be mutually voluntary or should become voluntary early in the process of working through.

2. The definition of *client* should include those who will need to be influenced to achieve the desired outcome and maintain it.

Some Skills Utilized

Consultants may have the most appropriate and clarified values of our profession, but without development of appropriate skills to articulate and implement values we cannot afford to feel proud of them. *One of the most critical values of all* is to take the responsibility to develop the behavioral skills of effectively representing and expressing our values in action. In the little decision case previously discussed, these skills included

1. The skill of communicating the value rationale to the administrator so he did not feel threatened, accepted the rationale, and accepted the idea that the consultant "knew what he was up to and could pull it off"

2. The skill of meeting separately or together with the unit heads to support open communication about the problem situation and to elicit their readiness to work on it

3. The skill of projecting the kind of work that would be needed and getting support and sanction for working with the unit staffs

Decision 2. What and When Shall I Advocate?

The Situation. The board is in the process of setting 2-year goals that I feel are too ambitious (i.e., not feasible of accomplishment in that period), neglect to examine the probable duplication of services with interdependent agencies, and have some potentially very harmful results in terms of neglected clients and wasted United Way funds.

The Decision Dilemma

Shall I tell them what goals I believe are reasonable and advocate collaborative interaction with the other agencies, or will I be abdicating my consultant role if I "tell them what they ought to do"?

Some Decision-Action Alternatives as I See Them

1. Present my recommendations by being an advocate for my position (i.e., belief)

2. Present my ideas as another alternative for them to consider

3. Recommend problem-solving procedures I think will help them discover alternatives and consequences

4. Help them work on goals they have chosen, no matter how I feel about them

5. Decide that their values are incompatible with mine and I should withdraw from helping

6. Other alternatives?

Value Criteria I Feel the Need to Consider and Use

1. Every client has the right and responsibility to make his or her value decisions (i.e., goals).

2. But the consultant has the responsibility for helping the client use problem-solving methods and resources that are as appropriate as possible in making such decisions and plans.

3. The consultant should hold the idea that differences of value are normal and that the feeling that "they should believe like me" is a trap to which consultants must be sensitive.

4. If I feel my clients' behavior is going to be harmful to themselves or others, I may need to mobilize resources beyond my own to prevent damage.

5. Some other criteria you might consider?

The Decisions and Actions of This Consultant

1. I proposed two steps in goal setting, the first, brainstorming all possible desirable outcomes or goal images and the second, a prioritizing exercise that included feasibility testing by projecting the action steps required to get to the 2-year goal images.

2. I added my own items as part of the brainstorm.

3. I role played other agency directors reacting to their goal ideas and recommended some data collection (i.e., involvement of the others) as part of the final goal-setting process.

4. I raised questions about motivation and value issues when there was resistance in the form of a complaint of "paying too much attention" to how the other agencies would be affected by the goal decisions and plans.

5. I decided to continue as a consultant in spite of several decisions with which I disagreed.

Some Value Principles Utilized

1. There is a basic difference between *positional advocacy* and *methodological advocacy*, that is, between telling them what they should believe or do (or what I think they should believe or do) and what problem-solving methods I believe they should use.

2. Development and utilization of values and skills is a stepwise process. Expecting them to be "perfect," or the way I think they ought to

function, at any given point in our relationship is an unrealistic trap for my being helpful in stepwise development.

3. The helper has the responsibility for sharing his/her own perspectives as a resource, but in a shared problem-solving context rather than a dependency-creating or expert status-wielding mode.

4. The consultant may need to be ready to announce a decision to terminate the contract if he/she feels that collaborating in the activities has become a basic violation of ethical values that the client is unwilling or unable to consider issues to work on (i.e., clarify, revise, etc.).

Some Skills Utilized

1. The skill of making a credible presentation of the value of brainstorming alternatives and testing consequences

2. The methodological skill to lead such an activity if it is accepted

3. The skills and sensitivity to roleplay those who are not present without creating defensiveness

4. The skill of sharing own beliefs without giving them a central authority weight in problem solving.

These are all skills that require practice with feedback, debriefing, and repractice. They are part of the discipline of becoming an effective professional helper.

Decision 3. What About Confidentiality?

The Situation. I am meeting with the administrator of a community mental health facility where the staff is demoralized by some impending budget cutback decisions that will curtail valued programs and drop some personnel. The board at its last meeting has expressed displeasure at the evidences of staff discontent and the way the director is handling the situation. The administrator says, "Off the record, I need to tell you something that's going on with the board chairman and some of his cronies that is really aggravating the mess I am in."

The Decision Dilemma

Shall I accept an off-the-record contract or intervene at this moment to refuse this kind of commitment?

Some Decision-Action Alternatives as I See Them

1. Accept the request for confidentiality

2. Interpret my "contract" with the total client system as requiring that I use my discretion about what is the best use of all data I receive

3. Agree to the confidence but indicate that I may want to get the administrator's voluntary release for me to use the data if I can see the value of this use and he agrees

4. Others you might see?

The Value Criteria I See the Need to Consider and Use

1. Must not get into trap of having important data that would help in my consultant problem-solving role but not being free to use them

2. Must not support norms of secrecy that inhibit development of open feedback between the parts of the system

3. Need to be a trusted recipient of controversial data in order to make adequate diagnosis

4. Others you might consider?

The Decisions and Actions of This Consultant

1. I asked him if he would refrain from prejudging the best use of his observations, opinions, and feelings. I was committed not to do anything that would be harmful to his relations with the board and staff. After I heard the data I would recommend to him what I could see might be a helpful use of them.

2. After hearing his observations and belief about a clique of the board communicating with discontented staff and conspiring to oust him, I suggested I would like to have interviews with several staff and board members to get their assessments of the situation, indicating to them that I had already talked with him, with the idea of convening a problem-sharing session to give feedback on my perceptions of the problems to be mutually confronted.

Some Value Principles Utilized

1. Invoking of the confidentiality ethic is usually motivated by a need for self-protection or a distrust of others to make "professional" use of

data. This is usually dysfunctional to good problem solving or informed delivery of service.

2. To be loaded with the commitment to confidentiality may be to use confidentiality as a poor substitute for open communication.

3. To be perceived as a repository of confidential information can be interpreted as being in a role of advocacy or as "siding with" one party, leading to loss of credibility as an objective problem-solving helper.

Some Skills Utilized

1. The skill of inhibiting the natural personal inclination to respond positively to the offer of confidential sharing

2. The skill of helping the client see and accept the larger perspective of problem solving and the consultant's facilitator responsibility

3. The skill of convening distrusting, conflictual parties with a design and attitude that legitimizes the conflict of interests, communicates the payoff value of conflict resolution, and facilitates constructive, open communication

COMMENTS ON SOME DIFFICULT DECISIONS

These examples are just a sample of the important decisions that most frequently require thoughtful value clarification. This same approach should be applied to all the decision issues of the six phases of consultation.

Just a few comments on some less frequent but very critical decisions. No matter how thoughtful the contracting process has been, once in a while, the consultant finds that she or he has arrived at a point of basic incompatibility of values with the client. For example, even after an analysis of consequences reveals that the client's course of action will be harmful to others, the client refuses to consider goals and behaviors. In such a case the consultant must consider informing the client of a decision to terminate the helping relationship, must accept a responsibility to a larger client system, and must consider sharing observations of the danger with those who might be harmed.

Sometimes another basic dilemma emerges for the consultant, when he or she has to identify with one of two courses of action for the client: to adapt strategically to the norms and expectations of the larger system or to risk confronting the system and attempting to influence some change in it.

My experience has been that usually the job is first to help the client explore consequences and risks, second to explore whether the consultant can be helpful as a link to the larger system, and third to act as an affective and methodological supporter during risk-taking confrontations by the client. The key point is that the consultant continuously attempts to maintain the role of problem-solving supporter rather than problem-solution advocate.

QUALITY CONTROL SUPPORTS FOR ETHICAL BEHAVIOR

What I have tried to illustrate by this small sample of three decision situations is the type of internal dialogue I believe all consultants need to practice in order to gain competence in the development and use of value guidelines in the making of intervention decisions. None of us can or should do this aone. We need special help in actualizing our decisions in effective behavior.

What are some of our quality control and professional growth resources?

1. *Our colleagues.* Sharing decision dilemmas with colleagues is a sign of strength rather than weakness. It really is the initiating of significant leadership in one of the important areas of professional practice. Because such decisions must be made in interacting with clients, the best sharing and learning often comes in debriefing discussions when one is inviting reflection on decisions one has made and consequences one has observed. This has the effect of increasing one's repertoire of alternatives for "next time" and the clarity of one's values and their application.

2. *The professional society.* Most professional associations have had task forces or committees that have worked on a proposed code of professional ethics for membership. Some of these codes have gone beyond statements of virtue to illustrative case examples of situations and have recommended coping decisions and actions (Lippitt & Lippitt, 1978). It is very helpful to put on the program of association meetings dialogues and panels about current ethical issues.

3. *Professional reading.* It is easy to ignore exploration of value issues in favor of papers and books on new concepts and techniques of practice. But in every professional field there are a few colleagues who have a focus on values as a major concern. They are just as important innovators as other colleagues who are technique-focused.

4. *Self-inquiry.* Developing the skill of internal dialogue is a crucial aspect of our professional growth and of maintenance of a high level of practice.

One technique I have used for some years is to actually write, as a script, an internal dialogue between the voices inside me that are arguing or puzzling or comforting about a decision dilemma. I put at the top of the page the dilemma question or issue and then let the script unfold all the voices I can tune in on that have an opinion on the question.

The challenge is to take seriously the fact that in almost every professional decision made there are relevant and important value guidelines to consider and use, as well as technique guidelines and questions of the conceptual model of the helping process.

REFERENCES

Benne, K., Bradford, L., Gibb, J., Lippitt, R. *The laboratory method of changing and learning: Theory and application.* Palo Alto, Calif.: Science and Behavior Books, 1975.

Lippitt, G., & Lippitt, R. *The consulting process in action.* La Jolla, Calif.: University Associate Press, 1978.

Chapter 10

CONSULTATION AS A PROCESS
OF CREATING POWER
AN ECOLOGICAL VIEW

James G. Kelly, Ph.D.

When a consultant works on a mental health problem presented by a consultee and wishes to have a positive impact upon the consultee's organization, then the consultant works to create power. In order for the consultant to be effective, the consultee must be helped to be more influential in solving problems. The consultant helps the consultee in assessing and managing the resources—both latent and present, within and outside the system—that can be used to solve those problems. Power is defined by the amount of resources available within an organization and potentially accessible to the consultee. Creating power is essential for the consultation process, since the consultant, as an outsider, cannot bring enough new resources into the organization to make substantial improvements in the mental health of consultees. Without power's being effected within the consultation relationship, there is the risk that the technical help the consultant does provide will be illusory. It is the writer's view that rapport between consultant and consultee and attitude changes within the consultee will not be sufficient to help. Structural and functional changes related to the definition and uses of resources will be needed when a positive impact is desired.[1]

Consultation referred to in this chapter is conducted so that the consultee organization is able first to use and then to renew its resources. The consultation may be program, administrative, or consultee centered, but the work is directed to achieve mutual goals agreed upon between the consultant and the consultee. The explicit hope is that the content and the process of consultation will complement each other and contribute substantial effects that are useful and lasting. When the consultation relationship views lasting impact as a goal, then the topic of power comes under sharp focus.

The discussion assumes that power can be reciprocal, rather than derived solely from superior-dependent relationships, and that the development of resources within the consultee organization evolves so that different bases of power are relied upon by the consultant and consultee (Emerson, 1962; French & Raven, 1959). The consultation relationship proceeds in sequence, with initial power expressed as a result of the consultant's technical knowledge (expert power). Then, with the sanctions gained at entry, the consultant works for more expanded influence (legitimate power).

At this point there is a directive force in the consultation relationship as consultees perceive the consultant acknowledging and providing rewards (reward power), complemented by the consultees identifying with the consultant (referent power). Although there is a logical possibility that the consultant's influence is strengthened by the use of another type of power— coercive power—this power is implied occasionally, but expressed rarely.

Thus there are numerous types of power. One important task of the consultant is to consider and develop the framework for the various elements of power important in the consultation. The number and types of power appropriate to utilize will vary from one setting to the next.

The amount of power available to the consultant at any one time is the amount of resources that the consultant has available at his or her disposal. The creative task in consultation is to direct this power in order to bring about a more positive quality of life within the organization and to assist the adaptation of the consultee in this setting. There is an explicit premise and normative value when developing the consultation relationship that affirm that a high-quality work environment encourages the personal development of its members as valued resources.

This chapter will focus upon steps that a consultant takes to improve the management of resources (power) within the organization. The consultant cannot give away power, but acts as a catalyst to help the consultee accomplish this development of resource utilization. Twenty guidelines will be presented for this development. First, attention will be given to 10 actions that can improve the availability of resources. Second, 10 actions will be cited that, if taken, can reduce constraints on the development of resources. The sets of 10 topics are complementary. Together the 20 actions view consultation as evolutionary planned change. They are offered to assist the consultant not only to survive but also to provide help that can be more lasting. This brief enumeration of guidelines is presented as a supplement to other discussions of consultation techniques (see, for example, Argyris, 1970; Baizerman & Hall, 1977; Blake & Mouton, 1976; Caplan, 1970; Kaplan, 1978; Lippitt, 1959; and Mannino, MacLennan, & Shore, 1975).

These guidelines are derived from an ecological perspective that the author believes can assist not only with assessment of the consultee organization, but also with design of the consultation process. The premise of the ecological view is to design interdependent relationships between persons and their social settings. The change process is mediated by redefining the relationships between members of the organization and their work settings.[2]

Developing answers to the following questions can illuminate the management of resources:

Does the consultant have a theory of social change? Is the theory applicable for doing consultation?

Does the consultant have a different view of people who have power than those who aspire to power? How can these views be reconciled?

Does the consultant know how to work with people who presently have power?

Does the consultant know how to work with people who desire change without communicating a false naiveté or secretly testing out the consultant's preferred Utopia?

Does the consultant appreciate how current ways of doing things help the organization? Does the consultant understand the time and energy involved when a new solution to a problem is developed?

Does the consultant have guidelines concerning when consultation is more useful and growth-enhancing than distracting and limiting?

Does the consultant have the calendar time and the personal and organizational resources to give to the consultee as needed?

The questions are basic and taxing. If the present writer did try, in earnest, to formulate answers, he would certainly give different answers when working with one consultee organization in contrast to another. The intent of the questions is not to provide a checkout sheet for the "good change agent"; rather it is to affirm that these questions are germane when creating power. Even if they cannot be answered satisfactorily, making an effort to answer them can give clues about the definition of the consultant role. Answering these questions will also bring to life the usefulness of the ecological analogy. From an ecological viewpoint, the consultant's task is to identify resource networks and to be active in stimulating new arrangements of resource networks.

The competence of a classroom teacher, for example, to manage and direct a child who is at the moment nonachieving can be enhanced when both the consultant and the consultee work out the solution by drawing upon the help of other children, other teachers, parents, and staff such as custodians, secretaries, and teachers' aides. The ecological point of view asserts that prevention of a person's health problem is achieved by involving available resources not now related to this particular topic and by identifying potential resources for the future. The consultant's competence resides in the ability to identify these local resources and then involve them in the preventive work. Particularly important, then, is the ability of the consultant and then the consultee to draw upon latent resources within the organization for solution of mental health problems.

The ecological thesis views persons and settings as interdependent: persons and settings mutually create opportunities and constraints. The ecological view asserts that inevitably there will be both negative and positive effects of consultative activity: the consultant is potentially both a help and a hindrance. In the consultation relationship, people, settings, and the change process are all viewed as resources to help social integration of the members of the organization and development of new competencies for the members. The consultation process is hindered when the accessibility of resources is incomplete and the consultant is unable to assist integration of members into the organization.[3]

Creating power relates to active efforts by the consultant to identify, then stimulate redefinition of, resources within the organization. Reducing constraints is redefining the social structures and social functions within the host organization that are at present preventing both people and settings from being resources.

Here are 10 guidelines for creating power and 10 guidelines for reducing constraints, to assist the consultant when developing impact within the consultee organization.

CREATING POWER

A request for help affirms that there is an incomplete or inadequate distribution of resources available for the consultee. The consultant's initial task is to make an appraisal of resources—while working to solve an immediate task. How the consultant goes about integrating and allocating resources when providing help will vary, depending upon the competencies and interests of the consultant and the operation of social norms for how an outsider works within the consultee organization. The following 10 topics, with brief commentary, are offered as suggestions for assessment and development of resources.

1. Identifying Individual and Group Competencies within the Organization

Many organizations are not aware of the resources that are available to them. Competencies of members include not only those technical skills needed to carry out the primary activities of the organization, but also leadership skills, personal qualities, and leisure time interests of members of the organization—not required for the performance of current work roles, but nevertheless potentially useful when considering the organization and its array of total resources. The consultant notes, acknowledges, and reaffirms these often unnoticed qualities and creates opportunities for them to be expressed. This is often and most easily done by casual observations and commentary, by making it clear, in an informal way, that the consultant considers these characteristics important. When such latent talents and skills have been noted by the consultant, then communicated to consultees, the consultant has taken a first step to test out the potential power of the organization, that is, its use of its resources. As organizations become more fragmented, employees often are less aware of their working colleagues, and consequently there is an unintended social tradition established that reduces opportunities for employees to note and benefit from each other and their settings. By "broadcasting" that these resources are present and available, the consultant observes how members of the consultee organization can take the initiative to benefit and to acknowledge these "natural" resources. As these steps are taken, the consultant notes how the organization creates social settings to celebrate these resources. By learning about them, the consultant has made an initial foray into the way resources are used.

2. Clarifying the Fit Between Means and Goals Across Social StatusGroupings

In developing a solution for a present problem and implementing that solution, the consultant accommodates to the existing ways the organization has developed to carry out its work. While going about solving the initial problem as presented by the consultee, the consultant can test out how solutions are implemented within the organization. This inquiry can lead to a clarification of how persons in the organization with different types of work roles perceive how the organization is achieving its goals and a clarification of how much potential is available for persons with different social rankings within the organization to agree on the means to achieve these goals. Any proposed solution for a current problem will bring into play differences between social status groupings within the organization. Social power is accrued to the consultant when the consultant clearly acknowledges what the consultees already know and live with every day: the fact that gradations of social influence operate within the organization. Development of a lasting solution to a problem will depend upon the commitment and the cooperation of persons in different status positions within the organization.

In addition, as the consultant identifies persons who can make alliances and create agreements across status groupings, the consultant is helping to define and develop the next generation of informal   leaders within the organization. If this reconnaissance goes well, the consultant is in a position to clarify for the consultees how latent resources are made available to the organization and can define the best ways for the organization to benefit from these resources.

3. Clarifying the Need for Long-Term Changes in Policy

As the consultee begins to solve an immediate problem, the consultant can assess how a new or modified policy, if implemented, can support the work that has just been accomplished by the consultee. This is where the consultant assists the consultee in evaluating the relative merits of one desired goal versus another and the merits of varied approaches to bring about an agreed-upon goal. The consultant balances an initial enthusiasm for successful problem solving with a matter-of-fact discussion of the merits and limitations of developing various long-range plans. A systematic, careful probing of the processes for policymaking can temper any unrealistic mood of change. An important distinction between the consultant and the consultee is not just enthusiasm to make a work environment a better place, but more important, theoretical and practical knowledge of ways to ensure that a good idea can be fairly evaluated. One criterion of the consultant's effectiveness is an ability to persuasively advocate that local resources be efficiently used and not wasted within the consultee's organization.

4. Creating Revisable Operational Procedures

As the consultation relationship proceeds and its goals are clarified, the need to design operational procedures and to take actions that will assist the organization emerges. Bylaws, policy handbooks, informal written agreements are examples of procedures to define what is intended, what is possible, and how the organization will transact its work. The consultant's presence and involvement in such activities can illustrate how new procedures can revise today's preferred ways of working. The consultees who are designing a new organizational charter can very easily become absorbed and preoccupied with the details of the document and the current dilemmas of the organization, and may not see how, for example, tight restrictions on the way work gets done can limit efforts at revising social policy or how, when specifications for operational details are too vague, frustration mounts over varied interpretations of "what is expected." Working to implement this guideline is recommended as an activity to help the consultee see the connection between day-to-day organizational activities and the drafting of rules of goverance.

5. Creating Social Activities that Can Help Members Identify with the Organization

Consultees, with their professional background and training, often have a condescending attitude about "cheerleading" behavior, that is, managing the social calendar. Yet the informal social occasions of the organization can help consultees not only identify with the organization but also feel integrated within their work environment. These informal occasions are interdependent with the design of rules of governance. An organization without rules will be anarchic and no doubt will become directly or indirectly self-destructive. An organization without informal social occasions will be sterile, potentially anomic, and at least dominated by social cliques. While going about the task of working on a current problem, the consultant watches for occasions to encourage celebrations and participation in informal talk and banter, which can soften the boundaries of official work roles. The more such occasions can involve representatives of all social strata, the more these informal activities can keep alive the social norm that the organization is using to improve the quality of the organization. Celebrations of good performance and social events help to solidify and validate membership and motivate people to become a part of the organization. When the consultant is alert to applaud such traditions, she or he affirms a value for the care and feeding of resources.

6. Creating Social Settings and Social Structures that Reduce Tension

Glidewell, in developing a conceptual framework for induced change, presented as one principle the need for creating methods to reduce tension (Glidewell, 1976). From my personal experiences in doing mental health consultation and in supervising consultants, I believe that this principle is essential for creating power. All organizations no doubt should create ways to reduce tension, but organizations that are developing a new service program activity particularly require methods to reduce tension. Without available ways to reduce tension generated while doing something new within the organization, the energy demanded by the organization for the change process can disrupt the consultant-consultee relationship. Social organizations that develop traditions to work through such pressures can be predicted to make better use of resources. The consultant assists with this essential task by first identifying persons who can take the initiative to reduce these tensions. The consultant's presence as an outsider can assist members to express their reservations in a controlled atmosphere where there is less opportunity for personal recrimination. An important facet of the consultant's role in this work is to communicate to consultees the validity of carrying out this guideline in a planned way. One way to reduce tension involves scheduling periodic occasions for people to express their views and feelings about the work, so that there is ease and a lack of self-consciousness in reducing tension.

7. Creating Support for Personal Growth of Consultees

As the consultee becomes identified with the solutions the consultant and the consultee have been developing, the consultee may become so involved in performing these tasks that personal development can be put aside. The consultant takes the initiative to hear what these plans are, is even solicitous about them, and encourages the consultee to pursue such plans and not become overly identified with the present work that happens to be in close collaboration with the consultant. The consultant works to reduce "trained incapacities" and communicates that the consultant has genuine interest in the consultee as a person and not just as a resource to the organization. The consultant also communicates a "gut" understanding about the risks of feeling "burned out" as the result of the taking on difficult or novel assignments. Preserving resources is as essential a part of the consultant role as creating resources.

8. Creating Communication with Outside Organizational Resources

This guideline affirms a second hypothesis of Glidewell's, namely, that the adaptive organization develops functional communications with other organizations (Glidewell, 1976). As consultees become invested in their work, a perception emerges that their work is unique and special. This "ethnocentrism" has a negative characteristic. It expresses the value that there are no other persons who can help, and that there are no other ideas that are useful, except those of the consultant-consultee team. The consultant exerts energy to reduce this fiction by giving attention to locating those persons and those organizations who are doing similar work and to evaluating with the consultee the benefits and shortcomings of establishing contact with such resources. A related issue is how well the consultant can assist the consultee organization to create reciprocal relationships with these potential resources. In many ways, the consultant is probing how the consultee can learn to work collaboratively without unnecessary competitive and exploitive motives. It is assumed that, when consultees learn to depend upon and trust other persons within *other* organizations, they can work to design a framework for long-range problem solving within their own organization. Once identified, these external resources can become involved in the work of the organization. The benefit of such new relationships is that, when collaboration becomes more explicit, the consultee then becomes more firm and clear about personal and role identities within his or her own organization.

9. Defining Support for Expression of Autonomy

Not all consultees will feel enthusiastic about the work of the consultant and not all consultees will share in the actual solving of the problem at hand. Nor do all organization members need to be involved with the aims of the consultation. One of the realistic anxieties of persons who are not initially a part of a consultative effort is whether they will be coerced into the new effort; they fear for their autonomy. The consultant is alert to ensuring that there *is* autonomy for organization members and that they can pursue their preferred tasks, even though at the present time these do not coincide with or relate directly to the aims of the proposed consultation. Autonomy is a special feature of individual growth and development, and members of an organization need to know that they have a right to autonomy. This point of view validates the consultant's assertions that consultees have autonomy to develop their personal interests and will not be consumed by a zeal to carry out the special and new work generated by the consultation relationship. The consultant gives particular attention to the views of the administrators within the organization who have given sanction for the work of the consultant. The topic of autonomy can be diagnostic of the administrators' values about how much autonomy can help the organization and how much autonomy detracts from the organization's achieving its goals. The consultant works to clarify the administrators' position on this issue prior to encouraging expression of autonomy among the other consultees. The consequences of this work are that the organization begins to see that differences are tolerated, that organizational work proceeds and does not consume others, and that there is an explicit value to help members of the organization be resources to themselves. Organization members acknowledge that the value for development is real even when being a resource means being independent of the consultant.

10. Reducing Seriousness within the Organization: Encouraging Fun

The tension and professional aura under which consultation takes place creates an unintended, negative consequence—an unnecessary seriousness. The seriousness can unwittingly stimulate a foreboding atmosphere. To lessen these effects, the consultant lightens the tone. A sense of humor can be a useful competence of the consultant when stimulating these softer and lighter moments. Noting humorous events, being able to reduce tension via laughter—particularly at the consultant's expense—is a skill that is appreciated and will be contagious. What is laughed at and enjoyed emerges as a unifying and motivating consequence of the consultant-consultee relationship. The consultant is then able to be perceived as human, too, and can loosen formidable attributes assigned to himself or herself. Making it possible to laugh implies that it is also acceptable not to achieve as much as was expected or hoped for and minimizes the negative effects of feeling incompetent when a problem is not solved, when the new innovation is not adopted, and when the efforts at the consulting relationship are not what was intended or hoped for. The professional veneer is washed off and is replaced by a shared sense of dignity about trying.

These 10 guidelines, these rules of thumb, have been presented to affirm that the consultant-consultee relationship can stimulate identifying, managing, and protecting resources. These guidelines can be tested to see if, when the consultant activates resources, the organization is helped.

REDUCING CONSTRAINTS

The following 10 guidelines are complementary with the first 10 and emphasize the consultant's need to help consultees and their organizations reduce internal obstacles related to the control and management of resources. Reducing such obstacles includes creating *new* relationships with other organizations, redefining present styles of communication with other organizations, and working to limit the negative feedback of undeveloped communication with other organizations. These guidelines focus upon the consultee organization and its potential array of new functional relationships. Successfully reducing constraints produces new relationships with other organizations, with the effect that the resources of the host organization can now be linked with resources of other organizations. Reducing the following constraints also makes it possible for the latent energy within the organization to be expressed, thereby creating new coalitions of resources. Here are the 10 guidelines:

1. Encouraging Consultees to Increase Personal and Social Integration outside the Organization

A constraint for many consultees is that they are not active members of a social group: they are either unconnected with a social structure or in the process of becoming disconnected. When an organizational crisis occurs they are vulnerable and seek outside help. Since the consulting relationship is demanding and produces its own stresses, the consultee will need to be a part of a primary social unit in order to limit the stresses of being a consultee. For these reasons as well as the intrinsic validity of the activity itself, the consultant encourages the consultee to become an active member within a social milieu outside the organization. To the extent that the consultee can be an active member within an external milieu, there is an increased chance that the consultee will be more of a leader within the work setting and a new resource for members of the organization. Working to increase personal and social integration of consultees reflects the consultant's awareness that it is not possible or desirable to be completely removed from the current personal status of the consultee. Although the consultant does not dwell upon this topic, he/she is attentive and acknowledges that there are more important features to effective living than simply becoming a better consultee. In the earlier writings about consultation, specific attention was given to maintaining a nonpsychotherapeutic relationship between the consultant and the consultee. The consultant did not focus upon personal concerns or issues that did not directly relate to the work role of the consultee—the privacy of the consultee was honored. I believe it is advisable for the consultant, while not probing for personal or family topics, to be alert for evidence not only of strains and tensions in the personal world of the consultees, but also of how consultees are maintaining or enhancing their integration with their surrounding culture. While not elaborating the nonwork roles of consultees, the consultant can encourage and acknowledge the consultees' other contexts, thereby indirectly strengthening general adaptation.

With an increased sense of personal and social integration, a consultee can be effective and influential within the organization as well.

2. Encouraging Development of Natural Support Systems within the Organization

A complementary preventive intervention for the consultant is to help the consultee realize the necessity of being a part of a number of socially supportive relationships within the consultee organization. Not only is it important for the consultee to feel a part of a social milieu outside the organization, as mentioned in the previous guideline, but it is equally important for consultees to feel anchored and valued in a social group within the organization. Consultees, trained in the human services, paradoxically are not aware of or do not admit their own personal needs. Consequently the consultant can be helpful in encouraging consultees, particularly those in human service organizations, to improve their personal connectedness within the organization. Informally drawing out the consultee and inquiring about the relationships that the consultee would like to strengthen, helping the consultee to have a clearer self-consciousness about current satisfactory and enjoyable work relationships, and encouraging the consultee to be explicit about the persons he or she respects and values can aid the consultee. The consultee then can more fully experience and appreciate the value of continuous, socially supportive relationships in the work environment.

Encouraging different types of socially supportive relationships is also important, so that the consultee does not become dependent upon any one individual or one social group as the dominant source of influence or help. If consultees do not feel recognized or valued, their ability to be a resource for others within the organization is reduced. Consequently they can end up going through the motions of problem solving in a mechanical manner. When other members of the organization see the discrepancy between philosophy and deeds, there is an added sense of being disconnected. When the consultant realizes that a particular consultee is unable to develop a personal social support system, the consultant works to include other consultees within the work plan and allows the particular consultee to catch up with being integrated. This process is essential before asking any consultee to take on more responsible or visible roles within the organization.

3. Encouraging Anticipatory Coping for the Organization

When working on a current problem, the consultant can inadvertently put aside the long-term operation of the organization. The energy devoted to the here and now may create an impression that the main and essential activity of the organization is the work going on now. The consultant's task, however, is to focus upon the contextual issues likely to affect the organization in the future, such as emerging economic, political, or social issues within the larger community. A criterion for effective consultation is whether the consultee has emerged into an effective resource for planning as the organization copes in its environment. Focusing upon relationships between the consultee organization and other organizations has an additional benefit of helping the organization focus upon its goals, policies, and ability to secure resources for itself. Assisting with anticipatory guidance is helping the organization develop an integrated identity as a planful organization. When the consultant helps the consultee in this activity, the consultant is affirming that resources within the organization are needed both for emerging opportunities and to withstand undue external pressures. The consultant cautions that available resources cannot be consumed wholly for internal matters of the organization, but instead can be partially allocated for coping with the outside world—where, in fact, the potential for activating future power lies.

4. Encouraging Members to Communicate with Consumers and Influentials

Reducing constraints certainly includes making it possible for persons in the larger community to advocate for the organization. This requires that the consultee organization take time to increase opportunities for its members to become acquainted with and link with persons who are outside the organization. The consultant affirms that the consultee has a responsibility to assume a role in the creation of a constituency for the organization. The consultant is also alert to giving consultees support as they communicate and ask for help from persons who are above them in achieved social power or below them in social status. Asking for help from such persons requires the consultee to be able to express his or her personal qualities in these transactions and not rely only on the expression of professional roles. The role of the consultant is particularly salient in anticipating how the expression of personal qualities can conflict with organizational values. The consultant here again can draw out the consultee and discuss the conflicts that will emerge currently and potentially as the consultee asserts his or her uniqueness. The consultee's new role must be a compromise between how he or she wishes to be and how the organization really is. The consultant's awareness about the processes involved in generating policy changes can assist the consultee to make a better adaptation without merely adjusting to organizational values. The consultant is definitely attentive to making it possible for the consultee to initiate and realize choices in the performance of his or her work. Putting aside professional roles and expressing personal opinions and beliefs in an open manner documents that the consultee has taken a tangible step at creating power: helping to adopt new styles of communication with new resources. The consultee is then ready to assess the potential of affiliating with resources previously unknown to the organization.

5. Helping Identify Tangible Criteria for Acceptable Performance

In many organizations there is a tendency for people to act upon implicit goals, to rely on a general understanding of the criteria by which they are to be evaluated for what they do. To the extent that such criteria are ambiguous, they do not help bring clarity to the organization. As the consultant works within the organization, time is devoted to identifying how the organization can be more explicit about what is expected of its members. In human service organizations, there can emerge a perception that being explicit is being arbitrary. Presenting deadlines, requesting that work be performed by a certain date, or informing staff of specific expectations held for how work is to be performed can be awkward occasions because so often members of human service organizations have not had opportunities to make distinctions between being clear and being arbitrary and between being direct and being coercive. Being able to learn how to express these distinctions is of major importance in achieving influence. The consultant can be of help with this subtle yet essential topic by assisting consultees to be competent in making these distinctions. Without a clear set of working ideas for what is acceptable and unacceptable, members of the organization are uncertain about what resources are available and which resources are needed. The organization can then drift into an ineffective use of resources. Development of explicit criteria for performance also helps organization members recruit citizens to assist the organization with the next series of activities. As the consultant works to help consultees be more explicit, there are also new opportunities to help members of the organization be more explicit about how they relate to each other as they do their work. Being explicit includes demonstrating how each member can help other members within the organization.

6. Developing Public and Explicit Criteria for Proposed Changes within the Organization

This guideline is complementary to the previous guideline. It refers to being open about how any proposed changes are stimulated by the consultation. As the consultation begins to take hold, as the consultant gives advice and offers help, and as the consultee begins to implement the consultant's suggestions, a threat is created from the very success. Other members of the organization begin to observe effects. They wonder what is transpiring and how this change is occurring. Most people have an intuitive sense of the difficulties involved when initiating personal or organization change, whether the changes relate to doing daily routines or learning new skills or adopting new ideas. When members of the organization observe directly a change in performance by one of its members, they are intrigued and wonder how it is being produced. They may even privately wish to be a part of it. Here the consultant does not allow much ambiguity to pervade. There is a benefit for the entire organization as the consultee and the consultant brief members about the consultation work undertaken so far. Such discussions and appraisals can be occasions for others within the organization to begin to take part. Being explicit also helps the consultant and the consultee to test their own ideas about what has worked and not worked. Most important, such discussions provide an opportunity for the consultation relationship not to be confused with any ongoing debates about preferred ways of carrying out the organization's work. Whether or not the consultant prefers it to occur, it is likely that members will cite the work of the consultant to support or refute their own preferred views on current internal debates.

By being public and explicit about what has been attempted, the consultant is able to maintain distance from ongoing debates and point out that the consultation process has an identity, a clarity and style, and goals that can be evaluated independently of other themes in the organization. Then the consultant gives opportunity for the ongoing debate to be redefined. The success of the consultant in asserting just how the consultation program overlaps and is congruent with, yet different in purpose and style, from other activities within the organization can present any factions within the organization, if factions exist, with the awareness that *neither* faction can fully embrace or claim the consultation program as supporting or confirming its own position. The consultant has then produced a subtle but palpable social force, so that both factions must consider other criteria that are producing their differences, including the possibility that the motivations for maintaining the factions are not helpful to the organization. The consultant, by example, asserts that conflicts cannot be clarified by simply identifying and claiming the consultant as either "ours" or "theirs." At least the consulting work will not be directly subverted as members work through these basic issues.

7. Conceptualizing the Consulting Process and Sharing it with the Consultees

A major role of the consultant is to develop a conceptual framework for the consulting process and then to express this understanding with consultees. When this is done, consultees can more assuredly learn new

168   THE MENTAL HEALTH CONSULTATION FIELD

ways to be resources within the organization. The consultant's ability to conceptualize the consultation process not only more clearly defines the relationship between consultant and consultee, but also gives the consultant and the consultee an opportunity to define how additional resources can be created within the organization. Since creating resources is a difficult task, being able to work with consultees and develop a shared concept for resource definition and resource management can clarify relationships between individual performance and the development of resources. When consultees realize that there is a direct relationship between what they do and how resources can be created, then the consultant is beginning to have impact. Consultees then possess a working perspective for how resources are defined and how the interconnection of resources contributes to a clearer and shared sense of organizational purpose.

8. Working So that New Ideas Can Be Adopted within the Social Norms of the Organization

Developing this guideline is often an elusive and neglected component of the consultant's work. When this guideline is implemented, it is possible to see the organization evolve and be responsive to future ideas and opportunities. When this particular guideline is not implemented, the change process stops. The task for the consultant is to arrange with key members of the organization so that new ideas can be tested and appraised. Here it is particularly important for representatives of the major units of the organization to evaluate and be able to accommodate to new ideas. This procedure is implemented to prevent creation of false dichotomies where, for example, those who are for change are "good" and those who are against change are "bad." It is the writer's observation that those members of an organization who question new ideas can over time be the most committed and involved members of the organization. They appear to value the organization to such an extent that they do not wish any outsider to limit or upset its structure. The consultant's ability to help consultees dissipate stereotypes about other members of the organization and to consider members' legitimate right to request serious appraisal can activate a force in the organization and make it more difficult for members to become divided against each other over any intended new ideas. The consultant determines just how different parts of the organization can be involved in the evaluation of a new idea and how the organization can create an evaluation process to see if in fact a new idea *is* a new resource.

9. Improvising Social Settings and Social Occasions to Stimulate Renewal

One of the characteristics of professional work is that it be explicit, orderly, and goal directed. This is true to a point. If professional work is carried out doggedly, it will prevent the organization from working in an informal and relaxed style and reduce chances for new ideas to be considered. The consultant's ability to improvise, to take advantage of ongoing activities and events, and to deviate from the plan—from time to time—will make it possible for the consultant and the consultees to experience the benefits of trial and error—to make a stab at doing something different and see if it will work. Both those desiring change and those skeptical of change will benefit from those occasional times to bring to the organization a new idea. It is not always possible to appreciate the validity of a major idea unless there is a chance to vary its implementation and make it possible for all concerned to weigh the opportunities and responsibilities for launching new ideas and to experience directly the pros and cons of a new procedure. Taking this step can also reduce a heavy professional air and temper the seriousness of the work. Here the consultant suggests how the organization can solve problems without a consultant, namely, to take time off from a work regime, select an alternative set of ideas and procedures, and work on clarifying the alternative ideas in an atmosphere of alert but relaxed understanding. The consultant can help achieve respect for the consultee and the members of the organization by providing examples of how resources are created.

10. Taking Advantage of Unplanned Crises

A complement to improvising daily activities is taking advantage of major unplanned crises to help create new social norms within the organization. In the author's personal experience, the insights of Erich Lindemann and Gerald Caplan (Caplan, 1970) have been validated time and time again: at a time of crisis people are able to change. The consultant helps the consultee plan and work out the details of problem solutions that include development of new criteria for the use of resources, but the consultant is also able to move with speed to help the organization unify at a time of crisis. Up until the time of crisis, the consultant has helped create a conceptual framework within which the organization could define the tasks for problem definition and problem solution. The occasion of a crisis creates an opportunity for new ideas, new concepts to be accepted. Being able to mobilize existing resources at a time when the organization is experiencing stress is an essential hallmark of an effective consultant. Few of us wish for crises; we do not seek them. Yet when they occur they are often essential if not pivotal occasions for change activities to take place. The opportunity provided by a crisis makes it possible for the consultant to unify new social forces within the organization.

CONCLUSIONS

Twenty guidelines have been presented to assist the consultant in creating resources within the organization. The consultant, as an outsider, initially works to solve an immediate problem and then works to strengthen the organizational resources to solve future problems. To work for lasting impact is indeed difficult. Not to do so implies that the consultant is available to work for only transitory, even illusory effects. These guidelines are presented to help the consultant survive while stimulating the consultee organization to better understand, appraise, and, if needed, rearrange its resources.

The ecological analogy has been used to generate these ideas and to demonstrate the relationship between the management of resources and the creation of power. The ecological analogy affirms that the creation of power can be achieved as consultees develop new social relationships, new professional competencies, and new criteria for communicating with other organizations. When the consultant works to redefine and conserve resources, the members of the organization are in a position to evaluate their individual and collective performance when contributing to an evolving organization.

REFERENCE NOTES

1. The development of the ideas in this chapter has benefitted from the careful, critical review of Benjamin H. Gottlieb and the pointed and clarifying suggestions about creating power given to me by John C. Glidewell. Their help has improved both the elements of the presentation and the thinking that went into the presentation.

2. The ideas in the statement were developed while the author was a Fulbright Guest Professor, University of Osnabrück, Federal Republic of Germany. Appreciation is expressed to Gudrun Chafik of Fachbereich 3, University of Osnabruck, who typed the drafts and the final manuscript with diligence, quality, and speed.

3. The writer has presented the ecological analogy in previous publications. The following references bear most directly on the ideas presented in this chapter: Kelly (1968), Trickett, Kelly, and Todd (1972), Kelly (1977), and Kelly (1979).

REFERENCES

Argyris, C. *Intervention theory and method.* Reading, Mass.; Addison-Wesley, 1970.

Baizerman, M., & Hall, W. T. Consultation as a political process. *Community Mental Health Journal,* 1977, *13,* 142-149.

Blake, R. R., & Mouton, J. S. *Consultation.* Reading, Mass.: Addison-Wesley, 1976.

Caplan, G. *The theory and practice of mental health consultation.* New York: Basic Books, 1970.

Emerson, R. M. Power-dependence relations. *American Sociological Review,* 1962, *27,* 31-41.

French, J. R. P., Jr., & Raven, B. The bases of social power. In D. Cartwright (Ed.), *Studies in social power.* Ann Arbor, Mich.: University of Michigan Press, 1959, pp. 150-167.

Glidewell, J. C. A theory of induced social change. *American Journal of Community Psychology,* 1976, *4,* 227-239.

Kaplan, R. E. Stages in developing a consulting relation: A case study of a   long beginning. *Journal of Applied Behavioral Science,* 1978, *14,* 43-60.

Kelly, J. G. Towards an ecological conception of preventive interventions. In J. W. Carter, Jr. (Ed.), *Research contributions from psychology to community health.* New York: Behavioral Publications, 1968.

———. Community psychology: Ecological approach. In B. B. Wolman (Ed.), *International encyclopedia of psychiatry, psychology, psychoanalysis, and neurology* (Vol. 3). Boston: Aesculapius, 1977.

———. 'Tain't what you do, it's the way that you do it. *American Journal of Community Psychology.* 1979, *7,* 244-261.

Lippitt, R. Dimensions of the consultant's job. *Journal of Social Issues,* 1959, *15,* 5-12.

Mannino, F. V., MacLennan, B. W., & Shore, M. F. *The practice of mental health consultation.* New York: Gardner Press, 1975.

Trickett, E. J., Kelly, J. G., & Todd, D. M. The social environment of the high school: Guidelines for individual change and organizational redevelopment. In S. Golann & C. Eisdorfer (Eds.), *Handbook of community mental health.* New York: Appleton-Century-Crofts, 1972.

Part IV

EVOLUTION

Chapter 11

THE EVOLUTION OF CONSULTATION

Saul Cooper, M.A.
William F. Hodges, Ph.D.

The major purpose of this section is to look ahead to the future of mental health consultation. As we examine the three chapters, we can see that case consultation is more frequently described as part of our past rather than part of our future. We seem to be moving toward a systemic approach, and as we do so, we must reconsider our knowledge base very carefully. With movement toward a systemic approach, careful consideration will have to be given to sanctions available for and against consultation practitioners as they engage in what might be defined by some as *social engineering*. All systems are inevitably embedded in a political context, and political decisions are frequently intertwined with power distribution. Therefore one major question we must address relates to the willingness of communities to give sanction for systemic consultations that might in fact impact on the distribution of power. What rewards can be offered to communities to allow systemic interventions? Although the ''competent community'' (Iscoe, 1974) is fondly to be desired, do we have any assurances that opinion leaders in communities truly stand for competency and coping skills for all community members? One might suspect that the values and philosophy of consultants and mental health practitioners generally might well be at odds with those of the community opinion leaders.

The philosophical and value issues surrounding a movement toward systemic consultation must be carefully addressed if effective interventions are to be designed. The community funding source has obvious power to impact if it so chooses or to prevent change if it sees the present power distribution to be in its best interests. The consultant who wishes to effect systems changes in a community must operate from a power base within

the community, based on a history of trust, mutual benefit, and competence. Such a task of community change not only is complex and extremely
time-consuming but also may not in fact be technically possible in the
immediate future (if at all).

The history of the mental health field seems to suggest that, as long as
mental health practitioners deal with "deviancy" (as defined by community opinion leaders), then we will be allowed to function. Focusing on
organizations and systems from a publicly funded base, however, may not
be received kindly in most communities. The mental health consultant may
better understand his/her constraints if he/she recognizes that the history of
community-defined social deviancy in this country is almost identical with
the history of the mental health field. Extrusion, not assimilation, has been
the prevailing intervention of choice. The mental health "ghetto" of post
hospitalized patients has characteristics remarkably similar to the
characteristics of ethnic "ghettoes" both past and present. Despite the
concerns we have just expressed, we believe that the full impact of mental
health consultation will not be felt unless and until one moves toward a
systemic strategy in delivering consultation services. The history of the
mental health field forcefully highlights the direction of future research and
technology development that must be pursued by those senior consultants
with secure organizational bases and with the ability to conceptualize and
test out problem-solving approaches of a systemic nature. We believe that
the future positive impact of mental health consultation and the choice of
community arenas are inextricably linked.

INFORMAL SUPPORT SYSTEMS

Gottlieb makes some beginning differentiations between mutual-help
groups, natural helping networks, and informal support systems. The differentiations are vital if useful work is to be done in this area. The recent
literature on helping networks suggests a lack of clarity and considerable
confusion about definitions. Not all consultants may agree with the
Gottlieb distinctions, but Gottlieb certainly makes explicit one such set of
definitions, and at this point in our development he offers us a clearer way
of communicating with each other as we attempt to increase our knowledge
and build skills. We take seriously Gottlieb's cautions about the role of the
consultant with helping networks and we urge all consultants to be quite
sensitive to the issues he raises. We hope, however, that consultants will not
shy away from working with such networks, but instead will rather carefully design interventions that detect and enhance the natural development
of these networks.

One must put special emphasis on the cultural and ethnic issues that arise around helping networks. The essentially middle-class white background of most consultants puts them at a disadvantage in dealing with many support systems that have a strong cultural or ethnic base. We do not suggest that one must be part of an ethnic group in order to consult successfully with it, but the lack of sensitivity to cultural and ethnic issues can be most destructive to natural helping networks. Gottlieb most graphically underscores the issue when he talks about "colonizing indigenous helping arrangements."

Those consultants who see themselves as community psychologists are well aware of the "professional authority versus experiential authority" differentiation. The mental health consultant who comes out of a clinical background may not yet be fully sensitive to this differentiation. A systemic orientation assumes that experiential authority carries a certain degree of community legitimacy. Unless the consultant accepts this concept, he/she will be less than helpful with natural support systems. These two types of authority represent an almost universal backdrop to all human service transactions. We would suggest that a successful outcome is highly correlated with a resolution of the systemic tension generated between professional and experiential authority.

Gottlieb suggests that we must enhance the "mastery" aspirations of mutual-help groups. This once again raises value issues. Albee, Kelly, and others have exhorted those of us who are community psychologists to "give away" our expertise. Perhaps no less should be asked of the mental health consultant working with mutual-help groups. The process of giving expertise away is not an easy one. Success demands an understandable and usable set of skills geared to the mastery requirements of the helping networks.

A review of mental health services over the last 5 years clearly indicates a steadily increasing legitimizing of helping networks at the community level. We note that the National Institute of Mental Health (NIMH) has stressed the concept of community support systems as a major strategy for deinstitutionalized mental patients. Although this particular thrust focuses on people with moderate to severe pathology, the overall stress on community support systems will help to legitimize those systems geared to lesser degrees of pathology as well. The community-support-system focus would seem to have a much greater potential for "normalizing" the lives of ex-hospital patients than our previous clinical approaches. It also spotlights a full range of consultee agencies and organizations that need to be approached by our consultation programs.

Thus as we broaden our perspective we note that consultation is not limited to helping networks made up of consumers or potential consumers of mental health care, but should also include programs for mental health boards and advisory councils, for neighborhood or block clubs, for health systems agencies, for child care coordinating councils, for child abuse councils, and for a myriad of other organizations that may or may not neatly fit the category of informal support systems or natural helping networks. Whether or not they can be categorized, it is the systemic emphasis of the consultation that must be underscored.

Those of us who have been involved in system consultation for any length of time have also begun to recognize that control, domain, and power issues are no less important in natural helping networks than they are in formal bureaucratic organizations. The "virtue" of experiential authority is not sufficient to eliminate many of the problems one sees in dealing with systems that are informal versus systems that are formal. Diagnosis and intervention with natural helping networks is much more complex and requires much greater skill on the part of the mental health consultant than may be true in one-to-one psychotherapy.

HUMAN SERVICE NETWORKS

Goodstein leads us through a review of human service networks and makes a compelling argument for a system model of consultation as the preferred strategy. A careful reading of his material suggests, however, that the individual-process model and the educational model should not be too quickly put aside and that, in the final analysis, the competent mental health consultant will need to pick and choose from among all three models in dealing with human service networks.

In our experience, we have found that many human service systems are interlocking in nature and that this requires special consideration on the part of the consultant. The police system in practically every community, for example, has by statute an interlocking relationship with the court system. The police set their primary tasks as detection, apprehension, and conviction, but they require activity on the part of the court system in order to complete the third step in their self-described goals. On the other side of the fence, the court system requires "raw material" in the form of clients, most of whom are brought to court through the police system. Further one finds, as Alinsky (1971) so clearly demonstrated, that the "oversupply" or "undersupply" of "raw material" impacts quite significantly on any given human service system. We are reminded of an example that happened several years ago, when the Chicago police found that their requests for increased wages were not being heard by the city fathers. They designed an interesting strategy to make their case. In essence, they decided to "enforce the law" and by so doing increase significantly the number of clients brought before the court. The clogging of the court system and its reduced ability to function made staunch advocates of the judges in helping the police get their salary increase. In another example, we saw a police department reduce the number of juveniles brought before the court to practically zero because of a major philosophical difference between the courts and the police around juvenile delinquency. The courts emphasized rehabilitation whereas the police valued punishment as a deterrent.

There are a variety of other examples of interlocking human service systems, and it behooves the experienced consultant to understand these interlocking relationships. A lack of such sensitivity could produce consultation activites that further exacerbate the problems between systems and therefore reduce the quality of client intervention on the part of such systems. We have seen instances where mental health centers have assigned one consultant to one agency in an interlocking system and a different consultant to the other interlocking agency. The communication between consultants was minimal, and as a consequence the intervention strategies ranged from less than complementary to markedly antagonistic.

Goodstein highlights another problem often addressed by consultants. He notes that consultees frequently define their problem by the nature of their request for intervention. Just as in clinical practice, we must develop skills to help consultees state the nature of the problem rather than request a specific type of intervention. At the same time, Goodstein's observation about consultant behaviors must also not be overlooked. The consultant who is limited by either skill or preference to an educational approach may well be doing a disservice to any particular human service system. It seems gratuitous but necessary to emphasize that the intervention employed must be related to the system diagnosis. Too many of our colleagues force system diagnosis to fit their preferred intervention approach.

A more recent development needs to be noted at this point. We have found a number of human service organizations asking for consultants to perform what appears to be a "system mental health checkup." It would appear that the systems involved are not asking for help because of a particular problem or difficulty but simply feel that it is good organizational practice to review their entire situation perhaps every 2 or 3 years using an external consultant to do so. To the extent that mental health consultants have the skills to do a system checkup, we would be moving a good distance toward a preventive stance around human service systems as well as human service networks. We are most encouraged by the potential in a system checkup.

FUTURE DIRECTIONS

Klein tells us that where consultation services are located organizationally within their own system may be significant for future development. We cannot agree more strongly with him on this matter, and we would urge consultants and especially directors of consultation to consider carefully the issue addressed by Klein. In the near future, the healthy growth of consultation services may well be much more a function of their organizational location and base than a function of the skills and techniques of the consultants themselves.

Klein's discussion of agency boundaries versus "natural" community boundaries must also be underscored. As human service agencies and health care agencies evolve, they tend not to limit themselves to boundaries identical with that of the mental health system in most communities. This fact forces mental health centers to deal with "real" boundaries in an "unreal" way. Once again, control and domain issues must be addressed among and between mental health centers offering consultation services if we are to be more useful to consultee agencies.

In summary, this last section focuses on the concept of *linkages*, that is, linkages between individuals in self-help networks, linkages between human service systems, and linkages between mental health centers and the community at large. The authors have attempted to identify some of the special problems that must be addressed, but in every instance the building of effective coping linkages becomes the theme. In some ways that is the exact and, from our point of view, the appropriate target of systemic consultation: building effective coping and problem-solving linkages.

In our judgment, a successful future for mental health consultation will require (1) a systemic approach, (2) a community/ecological emphasis, and (3) an active commitment to design intervention strategies geared to "social deviance." Anything short of this perspective will ultimately lead to the death of consultation as an intervention strategy in favor of newer, more innovative approaches. A systemic approach using the broad perspective of the community as an ecological environment would provide for the evolution of consultation into effective coping and problem-solving processes.

REFERENCES

Alinsky, S. *Rules for Radicals,* 1971, New York: Random House.
Iscoe, I. Community psychology and the competent community. *American Psychologist,* 1974, *29,* 607-613.

Chapter 12

OPPORTUNITIES FOR COLLABORATION WITH INFORMAL SUPPORT SYSTEMS

Benjamin H. Gottlieb, Ph.D.

This chapter describes two types of informal support systems in the natural environment—mutual-help groups and natural helping networks—and considers the actions and roles that mental health professionals can take to improve and enlarge such informal helping arrangements in the community. The chapter opens with the argument that mental health consultation is an inappropriate and potentially dangerous form of collaboration with informal support systems. Consultation is inappropriate because the social context and helping processes offered by informal support systems are unfamiliar to professionals and contrast sharply with the usual institutional contexts in which mental health consultation has been practiced to date. It is a dangerous activity because it risks supplanting the positive social functions that arise from public participation in mutual-help activities. The body of the chapter expands on the suggestion that mental health workers can bring to bear a variety of nonclinical skills to augment the work of these natural service delivery systems and that professionals can also play a role in creating mutual-help groups and in animating the formation of natural helping networks. In addition, current clinical practices that enhance the social support among clients are reviewed, with special attention to approaches that assist clients to maintain social supports following professional treatment. The chapter concludes by noting the absence of research on informal support systems among minority populations, citing only two studies that provide information about the Hispanic community.

MENTAL HEALTH CONSULTATION AS ANNEXATION

Anyone interested in the genesis of contemporary community mental health practice is inevitably referred to the series of monographs prepared by the Joint Commission on Mental Illness and Health in the late 1950s. Particularly instructive for the student searching for the origins of mental health consultation as a distinct mode of intervention is the volume titled *Community Resources in Mental Health* (Robinson, De Marche, & Wagle, 1960). That report documented the extensive role of such persons as teachers, clergy, and physicians in routinely providing support and a listening ear to the public. The report did not, however, reveal that these informal care givers mistrusted their own efforts to be useful to others, nor did it uncover critical sentiments on the part of those who had discussed their worries with these helpers. Indeed, the commission did not seriously inquire into the efficacy of the help extended by these community care givers, but proceeded nevertheless to issue a mandate for expert supervision of their work:

> Such therapy, combining some elements of psychiatric treatment, client counseling, "someone to tell one's troubles to," and love for one's fellow man, obviously can be carried out in a variety of settings by institutions, groups and individuals, but in all cases should be undertaken under the auspices of recognized mental health agencies. (Robinson et al., 1960, p. X)

Hence the commission cast the process of everyday interpersonal helping into a therapeutic paradigm, while the partners in the transaction were elevated to the status of *client* and *mental health counselor*. With the situation redefined in the professional mold, the commission proceeded to the task of ensuring that expert guidance and training were available to the mental health counselor, a task that called for the services of a new professional expert—the mental health consultant—whose job would be to

> provide on-the-job training, general professional supervision of subprofessional activities, and the moral support and reassurance found to be essential for most persons working with the emotionally disturbed or mentally ill. (Robinson et al., 1960, p. XIII)

Aside from the fact that the commission did not examine its assumption that care-givers were in need of upgrading, and aside from the characterization of the care giver as less-than-professional rather than as a parallel and complementary resource, the commission's recommendations amounted to annexation of one sector of the community's lay support network.

THE CASE FOR WITHHOLDING MENTAL HEALTH CONSULTATION
FROM INFORMAL SUPPORT SYSTEMS

Equally interesting is the fact that the commission did not reach out beyond this sector to other settings in which informal helping transactions were routinely occurring. The authors of *Community Resources in Mental Health* did not, for example, recommend that professionals establish consulting relationships with prominent mutual-help groups, such as Alcoholics Anonymous, nor did they inquire into the helping functions of voluntary organizations, block associations, or indigenous helpers who could be distinguished from other citizens by the informal advice, practical service, and referral functions they provided in their localities. Today we know a great deal more about the work of these lay support networks than we did some two decades ago, but the problems involved in developing professional ties to these natural forms of service delivery are more complex, and the complexity arises from the fact that, in their form and substance, natural helping arrangements differ dramatically from the types of helping situations with which professionals are familiar. We can best illustrate their unique character by contrast with the helping context in which community care givers operate. This comparison will help us to appreciate the factors that have facilitated creation of a consulting role with care givers and the factors that prevent the professional from forming such a relationship with lay support networks.

Since community care givers are representatives of the primary institutions of the community, in one way or another their job involves regulation of public behavior. They work within the norms and values of these institutions and presumably guide the behavior of citizens in accordance with these standards. In their social interaction with the people they serve, they do not respond as ordinary citizens or as neighbors or as friends, but respond from the perspective of the roles they occupy. The fact that a role relationship exists between the two implies that they are not social equals: one has greater control, authority, and influence than the other.

When this kind of role relationship is transformed into a helping relationship through a request for personal aid, the status differences continue to operate. Now the care giver is a helper and the person with the problem is the "helpee." The care giver discloses little about himself/herself, preferring instead to advise the helpee, provide a new perspective on the helpee's problem, or refer the helpee to another care giver or to a professional service. Given this structure to the relationship, several other points follow. The helper typically offers "talking therapy"; he/she does not offer material aid, provide concrete assistance, or take action in the natural environment to diminish or remove the source of stress faced by the helpee. The helper's assistance is available only during regular work hours (and, on occasion, on an emergency basis) and is usually delivered in his/her work setting. Finally, there is no expectation on either part that the helpee will reciprocate in any form (other than fee payment) the help that has been provided.

In contrast, lay support networks are ubiquitous in the natural environment and typically arise spontaneously, either because persons who share a problem recognize their common predicament and resolve to find a means of coping with it together or because one or more citizens are in a position to perceive common needs or tensions among people in a locality and find ways of meeting those needs through organizing exchanges of indigenous resources. Typically, status differences based on occupational roles or socioeconomic-class distinctions are submerged due to the leveling effects of their shared concerns, and the helping relationships that are generated are characterized by mutual influence and a reciprocal exchange of services. Access to the help of the collectivity is usually not restricted to any single time or place, and the means of help include material aid, concrete services, social support, and practical suggestions for problem-solving action that are based on "experiential knowledge" (Borkman, 1976). The norms that arise favor mutual reliance, long-term attachment, and consensual decision making. Each member of such informal helping networks is both the recipient and the agent of help, but some members may occupy more central positions in the helping network either because they maintain a wider network of contacts than other members or by virtue of their high referent power, which stems from the "experiential expertise" (Borkman, 1976) they possess.

In considering these contrasting features of the two helping situations, it is apparent that community care givers operate in a context that is structured like the professional's, whereas the form and processes that arise in informal support systems depart dramatically from the professional's enterprise. Indeed, it is precisely this match between the professional's and the care-giver's styles of helping that provides support for and legitimacy to the role of mental health consultant, whereas the generally poor articulation between professional and informal helping arrangements underscores the irrelevance of consultation as customarily practiced.

Cognizant of these differences in the two helping styles, the President's Commission on Mental Health recently adopted a much more cautious stance than its predecessor, the Joint Commission, toward professional interaction with social support systems in the community:

> Often natural support systems are invisible to professional scrutiny because the assistance given and received is qualitatively different from that offered within disciplinary frames of reference and is rendered

outside the structure of the human services agencies within which most professionals work, i.e., within the family, in kin, kith, friendship and neighborhood social networks; religious denominations; common interest and mutual help groups. Professionals need to affirm the existence and worth of these natural helping networks. Linkages need to be developed between these social and community support systems, including mutual help groups, and the professional and formal institutional caregiving systems. They should be established on a basis of cooperation and collaboration, not cooptation and control, and without disturbing the potency of their very different helping processes. (President's Commission on Mental Health, 1978, p. 208)

This excerpt is noteworthy not only because of the strong language expressed in the warning that professionals avoid colonizing indigenous helping arrangements, but also because of the expression of faith in the "worth" and "potency" of these supports. Moreover, the commission's optimism about the value of these supports is not founded on empirical evidence of their efficacy, since very little evaluative research has been completed, but is likely associated with two factors. First, the commission is aware of historical developments surrounding the genesis of many lay helping networks, particularly that the very origins of many mutual-help groups reflect efforts to fill the gaps in the professional service delivery structure and/or public dissatisfaction with the manner in which formal help is extended. Second, the commission's favorable posture toward informal support systems reflects recognition of the positive social functions that accrue from public participation in voluntary and mutual-helping networks. More detailed discussion of both issues—the weaknesses in the professional delivery system and the social functions arising from lay help—may clarify why professionals should pursue novel modes of inter-action with lay helping networks.

First, it is important to recognize that many mutual-help groups, the most organized type of informal help, have arisen as popular reactions to the weaknesses and gaps in the professional sphere. In some instances, they have evolved to meet the needs of troubled people whom professionals have not been able to serve effectively (e.g. alcoholics, abusing parents) or people who experience acute stress triggered by entering unfamiliar roles (e.g., new parents) or new environments (e.g., university freshmen), but who are not mentally ill as defined either by themselves or by existing clinical or epidemiological tools. Furthermore, less visible and less organized forms of lay helping networks have been identified in settings where human service organizations are unavailable (e.g., rural areas) or where the services that are offered are unacceptable because they clash with the cultural beliefs or ideology of citizens. In addition, numerous informal social support groups have arisen in situations where people do not define themselves as appropriate candidates for professional intervention, since they are not anxiety-ridden or suffering from skill deficits, but where they are seeking support for a deviant life-style (e.g., gay rights groups) or help in coming to terms with a chronic medical condition or addiction of a family member (e.g., Al-Anon, Association of Retarded Citizens).

Aside from their importance in responding to the human needs that professional services ignore or that they address in ineffective or unacceptable ways, lay helping networks are unique in generating certain desirable social functions. They enhance personal esteem through promoting an awareness that each participant can competently help others; they provide a "psychological sense of community" (Sarason, 1974) through attachment to a primary group that provides respect, support, and a feeling of belongingness; they normalize feelings of deviancy through the recognition that others experience similar feelings and personal doubts; as a helping enterprise initially composed of strangers but subsequently forming a cohesive collective, they can reach out widely and in a coordinated manner to identify new members; through their group work they are able both to mold and to adapt to a new personal identity, and they can redefine the public's definition of their situation or condition in a less stigmatizing direction; and most important, they increase the likelihood that future problems or needs will be resolved through informal auspices, thus strengthening people's faith in mutual help and decreasing their reliance on formal services.

To summarize, this chapter calls for new forms of collaboration between professionals and informal helping networks, forms of collaboration that do not rely upon the deployment of clinical skills on the part of professionals since these skills are not consistent with the means of influence and the helping context of informal support networks. Furthermore, as an extension of clinical practice, mental health consultation may supplant the social functions served by the mutual-help movement. Instead mental health professionals can call upon other skills, including their preparation in basic research, evaluative research, problem solving, and program planning, and apply them in activities directed toward extending the reach of natural service delivery networks. At the same time, professionals who are currently engaged in clinical practice can seek to enlarge the social support available to their clients both by referring them to appropriate mutual-help groups and by intervening directly to strengthen the primary groups with which clients affiliate naturally. The following discussion first summarizes areas of current practice that should be enlarged because they involve the creation or enhancement of informal social support among clients now in treatment. Then attention turns to the use of professional skills for the purposes of reinforcing and extending the activities of informal support networks in the natural environment.

PROFESSIONAL PRACTICES THAT ENHANCE CLIENTS' SOCIAL SUPPORT

This section reviews several forms of professional practice that can strengthen the social support available to persons who are currently in the formal treatment system. Two main approaches are discussed: efforts to enhance the quality of support within the client's *existing* social network and efforts to link the client to a *new* and supportive social milieu.

The *social network* is a term that refers to the people with whom an individual normally interacts on a face-to-face basis, including social intimates, such as nuclear-family members and close friends, and more socially distant persons, such as neighbors, co-workers, and extended-family members. Contemporary clinical practice includes various forms of therapy that stress the need to understand the behavior of clients as a function of the network of relations in which they participate and forms of therapy that adopt the network itself as the target of change. Variations of family therapy are outstanding examples of this orientation, and network therapy (Rueveni, 1979) represents an extension of the therapist's interest in modifying the nuclear family to include the entire social set with whom the client interacts regularly. A third example of approaches to modifying and strengthening the social milieu of the client was reported by Gatti and Colman (1976). Labeled *community network therapy*, this approach involves the professional in family therapy and as an advocate in the client's relationships with community institutions and care givers. The approach is particularly interesting as a "hybrid model," since, on the one hand, it capitalizes on the professional's status in the community and influence with its institutions and, on the other hand, it reflects a style of helping that is practical and congruent with the everyday language and experience of the citizens who are involved. Although Gatti and Colman use systems theory to plan the work of mobilizing social support on their client's behalf, their style of practice reflects the premium they place on professional flexibility in forming relationships with the people who are responsible for sustaining the client on a continuing basis in the community.

A second approach to mobilizing social support on behalf of those who have entered professional treatment involves creation of a new network of support rather than efforts to strengthen existing, but weak supports. The family cluster model reported by Sawin (1975), Budman's *psychoeducational groups*, (Budman, 1975), and Fairweather, Sanders, Maynard, and Cressler's community lodge program for ex-mental patients (Fairweather et al., 1969) are prime examples of this approach.

In the family cluster, four or five unrelated families meet periodically under trained leadership. The program is intended to serve primary preventive functions, allowing the members to explore family dynamics and values, and their relations with the broader community, all within a context that encourages mutual support and growth. The approach represents a mix of the values underlying T-group training and existential theology. Although it is initially composed of families from the same religious congregation and meets under pastoral guidance, the cluster is intended to be a continuing social support system in the community. Budman has adopted a very similar approach by using his agency base to identify individuals or families experiencing similar presenting problems or undergoing common life transitions. He then holds group sessions in which participants are encouraged to share their experiences and feelings and to discuss coping strategies. As the process of social comparison unfolds, cohesion and group identification mount and the frequency of mutual help increases. Once a supportive culture exists, the professional gradually withdraws, and the group eventually continues independently in the natural environment. It should be noted that Budman's approach, in turn, has much in common with the model of the *situation/transition group* developed by the Transition Center in New Haven, Connecticut (Schwartz, 1975). Indeed, that setting is devoted solely to the creation of support groups for people experiencing a variety of stressful life changes or novel situations. Its disadvantage, in comparison, is that it does not attempt to transplant the group to the natural environment. It also casts the professional in the role of group leader, but a great deal of care is taken to avoid attaching a "mental health" label to the group, since

> "many would feel stigmatized or offended by being put into this [mental patient] role; others would feel the expectations of the sick role, involving neediness, dependency, and personal deficiency, as onerous, irrelevant or compelling" (Schwartz, 1975, p. 750).

The program of Fairweather et al. (1969) for easing the transition of mental patients from a hospital to a community context also follows a two-stage process: sheltered training and practice in mutual support precede group reentry into the natural environment. It is based on the conviction that mental patients can best achieve independence from institutional resources if they are equipped with the skills that underlie mutual reliance and mutual support. The program stands as one of the most effective and cost-efficient strategies for managing community care of the mentally ill. The program also stands as a cause célebrè of professional resistance to new practice arrangements that create a helping culture among clients and that, therefore, require a shift in the role of the professional. Fairweather attributed agency reluctance to adopt the lodge program to professional staffs [who] would not accept the program which would allow more autonomy for mental patients, since granting such autonomy would require unwelcome changes in professional roles'' (Fairweather et al., 1969, p. 101).

CONTRIBUTIONS OF PROFESSIONALS
TO INFORMAL SUPPORT SYSTEMS

The preceding section reviews a number of interventions that can enhance the social support available to persons who have engaged the formal service sector for help, but the remainder of this chapter considers the skills professionals can lend to those helping arrangements that have arisen spontaneously and independently in the natural environment. How can mental health workers use the full range of skills they have learned in order to further mobilize and promote such support systems, without altering their basic character or encouraging their reliance on formal bureaucracies? To meet this challenge, it is necessary first to distinguish among two main types of informal helping arrangements since proper identification of each precedes a determination of action possibilities. Hence forms of professional collaboration with mutual-help groups and with natural helping networks are considered separately. The chapter concludes with a brief discussion of the informal-help sources unique to certain ethnic minorities.

MUTUAL-HELP GROUPS

Mutual-help groups, popularly known as *self-help groups,* are the most visible and organized form of informal support. In the most recent of three books devoted to the study of such groups (see also Katz & Bender, 1976; Borman, 1975), Gartner and Riessman (1977) estimated that, worldwide, there are more than ½ million mutual-help groups. Although there are minor differences among definitions of the mutual-help group, most authors (e.g., Katz & Bender, 1976; Borkman, 1976) agree that the membership is composed of *peers* who have convened on a *voluntary* and *face-to-face* basis and who offer *mutual help* in solving a *common problem* or meeting a *common need.* A number of typologies of mutual-help groups have also been offered (Katz & Bender, 1976; Gartner & Riessman, 1977; Levy, 1976), including an outstanding review by Killilea (1976) of 20 characterizations of mutual-help groups. Riessman (1976) and Hurvitz (1974) discussed several major differences between clinical practice and the mode of functioning characteristic of mutual-help groups, and Borkman (1976) discussed the tensions between professionals and the mutual-help movement in terms of a fundamental conflict between the ascendency of "professional authority" and "experiential authority." Case studies of discrete mutual-help groups can be found in three journals that devoted special issues to the topic (*Social Policy*, 1976, *7* (2); *Journal of Applied Behavioral Science*, 1976, *12* (3); *Prevention in Human Services*, 1982 *1* (2), and the *Self-Help Reporter*, published by the National Self-Help Clearinghouse,[1] is a lively newsletter devoted to disseminating knowledge and resources in the self-help field.

Global statements about the prospects for and promises of professional involvement with mutual-help groups are interspersed in the literature cited here. Only two publications concentrated on potential forms of collaboration (Baker, 1977; Gottlieb & Schroter, 1978); three others brought data to bear on the topic. One provided a provocative lesson on the "perils of partnership" between the staff of a chapter of the American Cancer Society and "Cancervive," a mutual-help group initiated by the agency (Kleiman, Mantell, & Alexander, 1976). Another presented the findings of a survey of 748 mental health agencies regarding attitudes toward the use of self-help groups (Levy, 1978), and the most recent presented the opinions of mutual-help group members themselves about suitable roles for professionals to assume in self-help group activities (Gottlieb, 1982). These papers, considered alongside the recommendations of the Task Panel on Community Support Systems of the President's Commission on Mental Health (1978), suggest a series of action guidelines for professionals seeking to maximize the role of mutual-help groups in the health-maintenance field.

Heightening Knowledge of Mutual-Help Groups

In discussions of relations between the formal and informal service delivery systems, professionals are frequently exhorted to mobilize mutual-help groups both during and following their clients' entry into treatment. It is argued that direct collaboration of this sort represents one way in which professionals can demonstrate their commitment to such concepts as the need to provide a continuum of care to clients and the importance of bringing environmental resources to bear on health-maintenance tasks. Indeed, much of the interest in community support systems expressed by the President's Commission on Mental Health was prompted by concern for the plight of mentally ill and recently discharged patients who have been indiscriminately "dumped" in community settings without the supports necessary to foster their social reintegration. Recent recognition of the link between successful community tenure and the availability of social supports has spurred the creation of programs such as Berkeley House, a psychiatric halfway house organized as an "extended psychosocial kinship system" (Budson & Jolley, 1978). Other agencies charged with the responsibility for aftercare and treatment programs are now actively collaborating with such mutual-help groups as Recovery, Inc. (see Wechsler, 1960, for a detailed description of this group) and Neurotics Anonymous. Similarly, workers in alcohol treatment programs routinely refer clients to Alcoholics Anonymous for concurrent help, and professionals involved with the mentally retarded suggest that family members join appropriate informal associations.

In order to effect a higher rate of professional referrals to mutual-help groups, certain basic problems that hinder productive relations must be overcome. On the one hand, the bulk of mutual-help groups are not affiliated with a large national organization and therefore do not have the funds or the personnel to advertise and interpret their functions to the appropriate professional and public audiences. On the other hand, the professional sector neither has been trained to consider mutual-help groups as a referral option nor is under any pressure from peers or from clients to do so. Under these circumstances the professional remains oblivious to existing mutual-help groups or comes to perceive them as irrelevant to professional practice. Levy's survey (1978) of mental health professionals' perceptions of the role and effectiveness of mutual-help groups provides documentation for this conclusion. When questioned about the importance of the role of mutual-help groups in the mental health delivery system, 36 percent of those responding said they were uncertain, and 39 percent were uncertain when questioned about the probability that such groups would become integrated into their agencies' service system. Perhaps more indicative of the professionals' general lack of knowledge about mutual-help groups is the fact that less than half the agencies sampled actually answered either of the two preceding questions, indicating to Levy that "they lacked the basis upon which to make an informed response" (p. 309)

A number of actions intended to increase public and professional awareness of mutual-help groups have been recommended in the hope that greater knowledge will lead to greater utilization. For example, the President's Commission on Mental Health (1978) suggested that all community mental health centers compile and disseminate directories of such groups; that each regional office of the National Institute of Mental Health establish clearinghouses to integrate information about informal support networks, to provide training and technical assistance to such groups, and to sponsor regional conferences to facilitate interaction among such groups and between them and the professional sector; that training programs leading to professional degrees in the health fields incorporate curricula that focus on the role of lay resources in the promotion of health. This last recommendation is modeled upon the work of Community Self-Help, Inc., an organization composed of people from a number of mutual-help groups in Toronto, Canada. Although its general mandate has been to educate the community at large about the work of its affiliates, CSH, Inc., has also focused on critical groups of health care providers. Workshops, for example, have been held with medical students on the use of mutual-help groups as adjunct treatment resources.

Improving Accuracy and Success of Referrals to Mutual-Help Groups

Campaigns to heighten professional knowledge about the existence of informal helping resources are not likely to improve the accuracy and success of referrals until professionals are persuaded that these resources suit their clients and work for them. A referral that is passed along only half-heartedly and is perceived by the client as an afterthought is unlikely to motivate the latter to engage in a novel and demanding treatment experience. Hence, to maximize the probability that a given client will act on a referral and profit from it, we need to inform the referral agent about such matters as the fit between the client's characteristics (e.g., stage of illness, ability to participate in a guided group experience, access to a personal support network) and the admission criteria informally established by the mutual-help group under consideration. Furthermore, since referral success is predicated upon communication of realistic expectations about the nature of the service or treatment the client will receive, the referral agent must be familiar with the details of programs offered by mutual-help groups. Indeed, mutual-help groups have as great a stake as professionals in research activities that can increase the accuracy of incoming referrals, since unacceptable candidates may communicate damaging sentiments about the group to the professional who originated the referral, whereas unsuitable parties may hinder group progress. Weiss's observations (1973) of the reactions expressed by and toward newcomers to Parents Without Partners testify to the need for empirical research on the characteristics of candidates who are best suited to participation in mutual-help groups:

> Nor is it easy to decide the sorts of individuals for which PWP will prove helpful. Some members describe the organization, with some exaggeration, as having saved their lives. Other single parents, whose needs would appear to have been similar, came to only one or two meetings and afterwards said they had been repelled by it. . . . The organization's ideology would require its members to welcome all those who are eligible, but in practice members respond more warmly to some than to others. (Weiss, 1973, p. 326)

To summarize, simply increasing the professional's knowledge about the prevalence of mutual-help groups is unlikely to increase the frequency, accuracy, and success of referrals to this sector of the community's informal treatment network. In addition, certain types of formative and summative evaluative research should be undertaken by community mental health workers in order to inform professionals and their clients about the processes and the impact of contrasting mutual-help groups. To date, detailed study of such groups has been undertaken largely through participant-observation and reliance on the personal testimony of participants. Antze's description (1976) of the ideologies underlying the work of three mutual-help organizations represents a good example of this sort of inquiry. The rich qualitative data generated by these approaches do not tell the whole story, however. In addition, survey research should be extended to this field of investigation so that more objective measures of the attitudes, health status, and behavioral change among participants can be weighed alongside the phenomenological evidence. Empirically based evaluative studies of the progress made by different types of people participating in diverse mutual-help groups can sharpen both referral and acceptance criteria while offering an agenda for self-study to the groups themselves. One excellent example of the utility of such evaluative research is the assessment of Parents Anonymous reported by Lieber and Baker (1977); a review of research on the effectiveness of Alcoholics Anonymous was conducted by Leach (1973). These sorts of studies can be undertaken by community mental health workers so long as they protect the anonymity of their respondents and so long as they develop a research partnership with the groups they approach. These activities also illustrate how professional training can be used to enhance the functioning and extend the reach of mutual-help groups without socializing them in the professional mold.

Professional Involvement in Creation of Mutual-Help Groups

Professionals can mobilize social support on behalf of clients who have entered the professional domain, either through directly intervening to strengthen their social networks or indirectly, by referring clients to mutual-help groups, and they can also become directly involved in the creation of mutual-help groups. There are significant precedents here, including the work of Abraham Low, a neuropsychiatrist who founded Recovery, Inc.; Leonard Lieber, a counselor who co-founded Parents Anonymous; and Dr. Bob, a physician who established Alcoholics Anonymous. More recently, Silverman (1970) and Mowrer (1972) created mutual-help groups for widows and "alienated" persons, respectively. Although the notion of a professional creating a mutual-help group appears contradictory, both Silverman and Mowrer were clear about the conditions under which professional sponsorship and involvement can occur. First, both the Widow-to-Widow program and Integrity Groups were launched from academic settings. They were not appendages of human service organizations and therefore did not conflict with the values, authority, and technology of a professional service system. As Silverman noted, serious problems have confronted agencies that have tried to deploy ''non-professional indigenous workers'' to mount programs similar to the Widow-to-Widow service:

> These non-professionals are usually given extensive training and supervision so that they begin to adopt professional values and emulate professional techniques. If they were following the self-help model, they should be making policy, developing their own techniques for helping, and the consumer of their services should be able to move into their role of caregiver. In the average agency setting this would be difficult to achieve since it would mean that the professionally-trained care giver could be displaced by his former client. He could also potentially lose control of policy as well as of practice. (Silverman, 1970, p. 547)

A case study of events leading to the failure of Cancervive, a mutual-help project undertaken by the Los Angeles chapter of the American Cancer Society, illuminates the struggles involved in operating a mutual-help group from a service agency base (Kleiman et al., 1976). Mowrer and Vattano (1976), however, believed that Integrity Groups can and should be mounted by community mental health centers, but they recommend that the professional sponsor withdraw from the group once it reaches a certain size. Similarly, Low initially decided that professionals should neither lead Recovery groups nor hold an office in the organization.

In short, professionals can play an important role in creating new occasions for the development of mutual-help groups by identifying and connecting people in similar stressful circumstances and by proposing a general scenario to be followed at group meetings (see, for example, McGuire & Gottlieb, 1979). The epidemiological tools available to identify high-risk groups—measurement of stressful life events (Holmes & Rahe, 1967), use of social indicators, and knowledge of critical life transitions—can be converged for the purpose of first identifying people ''in the same boat'' and then stimulating them to use the resources ''of the same boat'' and then stimulating them to use the resources of the collectivity for help in overcoming or accepting their situations.

NATURAL HELPING NETWORKS

Consultation and Collaboration with Natural Helping Networks

The term *natural helping network* was coined by Collins and Pancoast (1976) and designates an informal arrangement for the exchange of information, practical services, and emotional support among people who share a residential or neighborhood environment. Compared with the mutual-help group, the natural helping network is a less organized and less visible support system; it is not necessarily composed of people who share a similar problem; it does not call for its members to meet at regular intervals; nor does it espouse a single ideology about how personal change is best effected. Although a mutual-help group may evolve out of a natural helping network, the reverse cannot occur.

In their book, Collins & Pancoast (1976) provided several examples of natural helping networks, including a network of homeless men who frequent a tavern, tenants of single-room-occupancy hotels, and a neighborhood network that organized an informal day care service. Typically there are key influential individuals within these networks who can be distinguished from others on the basis of the personal and organizational resources they bring to the network and by virtue of their broad contacts within the network and in the larger human services community. Collins (1973) documented the pivotal role that such *natural neighbors* play in linking families to one another for the purpose of mutual help and in bringing external resources to bear on the needs of many families in their networks. Furthermore, she saw these central figures as appropriate candidates for mental health consultation with a focus on the provision of support and on efforts to enlarge the natural neighbors' reach in the community.

Specific guidelines for identifying natural helping networks and examples of the process of consulting with natural neighbors were published by Collins and Pancoast in a book that includes a variety of excellent formulations about ways of mobilizing natural helping networks to address problems of child maltreatment (Garbarino & Stocking, 1980). Donald Warren's chapter is especially noteworthy for its discussion of how neighborhoods differ in the informal helping resources they extend to residents, and elsewhere (Warren, 1978) he drew out the implications of his research for community mental health centers. He believed that novel programs are needed that capitalize on the existing pathways for resolving problems in different neighborhoods and strengthen their natural service delivery networks. He, too, identified neighborhood *reputational helpers* who function much like natural neighbors, and he recommended that mental health workers attempt to link these central figures to one another in order to strengthen their capacity to support people.

Warren's work was important because it identified structural characteristics of communities that are associated with varied patterns of help seeking and support, but his approach called for relatively sophisticated and prolonged data collection. In contrast, Garbarino, Crouter, and Sherman (1978) adopted a simpler approach to assessing neighborhoods as support systems for families. This approach provides information about the presence or absence of informal resources that bear upon specific types of neighborhood problems (e.g., delinquency, emotional dysfunction, drug abuse).[2] The research strategy involves application of a limited set of available social indicators, supplemented by a few survey items that are regressed upon a criterion reflecting the rate of occurrence of a given problem in several geographical areas. Using as an example the child maltreatment rates in 20 "neighborhood districts," the researchers found that five social indicators were excellent predictors of the actual rates of child maltreatment in all but 2 of the districts. These two had very similar predicted rates, since they were approximately matched on the five demographic and socioeconomic indicators, but their actual rates were very different, one showing a much higher rate than predicted and one much lower than predicted. Hypothesizing that in the latter case the discrepancy was due to the presence of active support networks among families, the authors surveyed a sample of residents in each district about their attachment to the community and their attitudes toward neighbors. The results confirmed this hypothesis, revealing negative sentiments among residents of the neighborhood whose actual rate was substantially greater than the predicted rate and positive sentiments in the locale whose rate was lower than predicted. Commenting on the overall value of this screening process for the work of child protective services, the authors concluded that "limited agency resources can be better allocated, the researcher integrated into the service system as a source of feedback, and neighborhood groups advised of likely targets for community action" (Garbarino, Crouter, & Sherman, 1978, p. 143). As noted earlier, this screening method can be modified for use in assessing neighborhoods for intervention on the basis of the rates of other mental health-linked problems; alternatively, rates of general utilization of mental health services can be adopted as the criterion variable. Zautra and Simons (1978), for example, identified 10 social indicators and a set of survey measures that predict mental health utilization rates at a high level of accuracy, and these measures can be used to identify geographic areas where the presence of natural helping networks can account for lower-than-predicted utilization rates.

Programs to Stimulate Development of Natural Helping Networks

Two programs have been initiated for the purpose of strengthening informal helping processes in the natural environment. In Guelph, Ontario (Canada), the "Human Services Community" (Bierman & Lumley, 1973) was originally funded by the federal government as a demonstration project in primary and secondary prevention. The program recruited citizens from three strata of the community—agency professionals, welfare recipients, and citizens inclined to work as volunteers in human service organizations—and offered them training in basic helping and human relations skills (Carkhuff, 1969). All participants who completed this first stage of training and who wished to proceed to advanced workshops were first required to teach the skills they had mastered to another individual. In this way the project could extend its reach more widely in the community while encouraging participants to view themselves as educators in their own social networks. Following this tutorial experience, participants could proceed to advanced workshops that focused on such specialized topics as methods of conflict resolution and adult-child communications. Advanced training was again followed by a period of service to the community in which the skills were imparted to members of the trainee's social network. The final stage of the educational program drew advanced participants into group leadership and training roles in the organization, thus ensuring a continuous flow of trained personnel to renew the learning cycle. Once a second generation of trainers was available, the small professional staff was freed to initiate outreach projects to vulnerable populations in the community. As examples, special workshops were extended to teachers in schools that served disadvantaged children and to single parents, while a program offering training in basic job readiness skills was made available to the chronically unemployed and underemployed.

The preventive thrust of the Human Services Community has been operationalized in two ways. First, it provides those basic helping and problem-solving skills that are deemed necessary to productive resolution of situational and developmental crises among its participants. Second, it ensures a systematic "spread of effect" (Bierman & Lumley, 1973) through a structured outreach program in the community. This outreach program involves the use of participants' training in direct helping activities within their own "personal communities" and in indirect service that takes the form of training others in basic helping skills. A detailed final report of the project, edited by Bierman (1976), contains impressive documentation of positive workshop effects on participants, as measured by a variety of standard personality tests and rating scales. Estimates of the program's cost savings are also presented but are largely based on speculations about the potential cost incurred had professional resources been used. The report also reveals the difficulties that attend evaluation of a communitywide campaign to build social support networks, and it reveals the weaknesses in this aspect of the program. Specifically, it was found that the outsiders who were tutored by graduates of the basic workshop did not significantly improve their helping skills (as measured by the standard pre-post empathy, respect, and self-experiencing scales), a finding that casts doubt on the program's ability to radiate helping skills in the broader community. Second, judgments about participants' success in reaching out to provide direct help to members of their networks were based purely on participants' self-reports about the number of hours they spent helping people and their satisfaction with the help they offered.

A second program, fashioned along similar lines, was implemented by a team of action researchers at the Pennsylvania State University (D'Augelli, Vallance, Danish, Young, & Gerdes, (1981). It, too, offers training in basic helping skills, encourages its trainees to pass these skills on to others, and offers advanced workshops in such "Life-Development Skills" as goal assessment, decision making, risk taking, and self-development. The unique feature of the program, however, is the way participants are initially chosen. The project's designers have attempted to identify and recruit persons who are natural helpers in the community and its primary institutions. They have attempted to reach out to these people by placing advertisements in the mass media, circulating brochures in public places such as the waiting rooms of agencies and medical practitioners, and soliciting names from members of voluntary and civic organizations. Their goal is to capitalize on the talents of persons who are currently engaged in informal helping activities in order to extend their repertoire of helping behaviors as well as their reach.

INDIGENOUS RESOURCES AMONG MINORITY CULTURES

Our review of the literature on mutual-help groups and natural helping networks has uncovered little information about ethnic group participation in such informal support systems. Our knowledge of subcultural preferences for informal support is limited to global statements concerning, for example, the importance of kinship ties and ethnic associations among Asian-American and Hispanic communities and the salience of the church and quasi-religious practitioners in the black community. Although we know a good deal about cultural influences on psychopathology (see, for example, Guthrie, 1973; King, 1978; Dohrenwend & Dohrenwend, 1974) and we have much evidence that minority populations underutilize mental health services (Rosenblatt & Mayer, 1972), our understanding of subcultural influences on help-seeking behavior is sorely limited.

A promising direction for research in this area is reflected in recent work on the role of spiritualists and other types of folk healers in the Hispanic community (Lubchansky, Egri, & Stokes, 1970). Ruiz and Langrod (1976) described the practices of such indigenous folk healers and their connection to the religious and medical belief systems of Puerto Ricans. Both papers explain how differences between the assumptions of modern psychiatry and those of spiritualists account for the resistance of Hispanic patients to medical treatment approaches, and both conclude with recommendations for collaboration between professionals and indigenous folk healers. The Lincoln Community Mental Health Center, for example, has produced a film that is used for training non-Hispanic staff, and the center has become involved in a productive referral relationship with the spiritualist temples in its catchment area.

A second approach to collaborative work with the informal care-giving network in minority communities was implemented by the New York Medical College (Leutz, 1976). Two staff members who were indigenous to the East Harlem section of Manhattan were able to identify 29 informal care givers, including clergy, merchants, spiritualists, and social club owners. The latter represents a type of care-giver who is unique to districts like East Harlem where, because of crime and urban renewal, commercial bars have disappeared and have been replaced by private social clubs. The owners are neighborhood residents who naturally become tied to the social networks of club members and thus become central figures in local networks of communication. Half the care-givers of each type were simply asked to keep a record of the contacts they had with people who were seeking help for drug-related problems, while the other half in addition were given a referral guide listing alternative treatment services for different drug problems. Each of the services was also discussed in detail with the "experimental care givers" in an effort to further train them in accurate referral practices.

The results of the study showed that the experimental care-givers referred more than 50 percent of the people who approached them with drug-related problems, whereas the care-givers who were not given referral information referred only 28 percent of the people who engaged them for help. Within the experimental group, the spiritualists and clergy proved to be the most active in referring people to treatment agencies, and the merchants and social club owners were much less active, a finding the authors explained in terms of the latter's financial stake in alcohol sales. The authors maintained, however, that social club owners carry a sizable "caseload," implying that if the study had concerned matters other than drugs and alcohol, these care-givers would have affected higher rates of referrals.

Taken together, both types of studies reviewed in this section suggest that unique sources of informal help exist in minority communities and that they represent expressions of sociocultural patterns, religious belief systems, or the popular culture among local residents. Agencies that serve these communities are advised to develop methods of identifying these indigenous resources. They should try to understand how they function and try to enlarge their work while preserving their cultural traditions.

CONCLUSIONS

The basic purpose of establishing ties with lay helping networks should be to further develop their potential to protect and enhance the health of citizens. Yet this goal must be pursued through avenues that do not foster dependence on a professional ideology or technology of change. Members of lay helping networks should be approached not as potential clients or consumers but as collaborators who have initiated forms of helping that they find useful and congruent with their own values and that they perceive as more acceptable than professional treatment. Recognizing that mutual aid is the hallmark of lay helping networks, professionals should seek to establish relationships that are characterized by the reciprocation of respect, skills, and knowledge. Although professional training equips the practitioner with multiple skills, it is less thorough in teaching about the selective use of such skills, and it totally disregards the circumstances under which professional expertise should be withheld.

NOTES

1. Free subscriptions may be ordered from the Editor, *Self-Help Reporter*, National Self-Help Clearinghouse, Graduate Center, CUNY, 33 West 42nd Street, Room 1227, New York, NY 10036.
2. Garbarino and Sherman described this technique in less technical terms in Garbarino and Stocking (1980).

REFERENCES

Antze, P. The role of ideologies in peer psychotherapy organizations: Some theoretical considerations and three case studies. *Journal of Applied Behavioral Science,* 1976, *12,* 323-346.

Baker, F. The interface between professional and natural support systems. *Clinical Social Work Journal,* 1977, *5,* 139-148.

Bierman, R. (Ed.). *Toward meeting fundamental human needs: Preventive effects of the Human Services Community.* Unpublished report, 1976. Available from Human Services Community, 23-25 Wyndham Street North, Guelph, Ontario, Canada.

————, & Lumley, C. Toward the humanizing community. *Ontario Psychologist,* 1973, *5,* 10-19.

Borkman, T. Experiential knowledge: A new concept for the analysis of self-help groups. *Social Service Review,* 1976, *50,* 445-456.

Borman, L. (Ed.). *Explorations in self-help and mutual aid.* Evanston, Ill.: Center for Urban Affairs, Northwestern University, 1975.

Budman, S. A strategy for preventive mental health intervention. *Professional Psychology,* 1975, *6,* 394-398.

Budson, R. D., & Jolley, R. E. A crucial factor in community program success: The extended psychosocial kinship system. *Schizophrenia Bulletin,* 1978, *4,* 609-621.

Carkhuff, R. R. *Helping and Human relations.* Vol. 1, *Selection and training.* New York: Holt, Rinehart & Winston, 1969.

Collins, A. H. Natural delivery systems: Accessible sources of power for mental health. *American Journal of Orthopsychiatry,* 1973, *43,* 46-52.

————, & Pancoast, D. L. *Natural helping networks.* Washington, D.C.: National Association of Social Workers, 1976.

D'Augelli, A., Vallance, T., Danish, S., Young, C., & Gerdes, J. The community helpers project: A description of a prevention strategy for rural communities. *Journal of Prevention,* 1981, *1,* 209-224.

Dohrenwend, B. P., & Dohrenwend, B. S. Social and cultural influences on psychopathology. *Annual Review of Psychology,* 1974, *25,* 417-452.

Fairweather, G. W., Sanders, D. H., Maynard, H., & Cressler, D. L. *Community life for the mentally ill.* Chicago: Aldine, 1969.

Garbarino, J., Crouter, A. C., & Sherman, D. Screening neighborhoods for intervention: A research model for child protective services. *Journal of Social Services Research,* 1978, *1,* 135-145.

Garbarino, J., & Stocking, H. (Eds.). *Protecting children from abuse and neglect.* San Francisco: Jossey-Bass, 1980.

Gartner, A., & Riessman, F. *Self-help in the human services.* San Francisco: Jossey-Bass, 1977.

Gatti, F., & Colman, C. Community network therapy: An approach to aiding families with troubled children. *American Journal of Orthopsychiatry,* 1976, *46,* 608-617.

Gottlieb, B. H. Mutual-help groups: Members' views of their benefits and of roles for professionals. *Prevention in human services,* 1982, 1 (2).

_____, & Schroter, C. Collaboration and resource exchange between professionals and natural support systems. *Professional Psychology,* 1978, *9,* 614-622.

Guthrie, G. M. Culture and mental disorder. In *Addison-Wesley module anthropology* (Module 39). Reading, Mass.: Addison-Wesley, 1973.

Holmes, T. H., & Rahe, R. H. The social readjustment rating scale. *Journal of Psychosomatic Research,* 1967, *11,* 213-218.

Hurvitz, N. Similarities and differences between conventional psychotherapy and peer self-help psychotherapy groups. In P. S. Roman & H. M. Trice (Eds.), *The sociology of psychotherapy.* New York: Aronson, 1974.

Journal of Applied Behavioral Science, 1976, *12* (3).

Katz, A. H., & Bender, E. I. *The strength in us: Self-help groups in the modern world.* New York: Franklin Watts, 1976.

Killilea, M. Mutual help organizations: Interpretations in the literature. In G. Caplan & M. Killilea (Eds.), *Support systems and mutual help.* New York: Grune and Stratton, 1976.

King, L. M. Social and cultural influence on psychopathology. *Annual Review of Psychology,* 1978, *29,* 405-434.

Kleiman, M. A., Mantell, J. E., & Alexander, E. S. Collaboration and its discontents. *Journal of Applied Behavioral Science,* 1976, *12,* 403-410.

Leach, B. Does Alcholics Anonymous really work? In P. Bourne & R. Fox (Eds.), *Alcoholism: Progress in research and treatment.* New York: Academic Press, 1973.

Leutz, W. N. The informal community caregiver: A link between the health care system and local residents. *American Journal of Orthopsychiatry,* 1976, *46,* 678-688.

Levy, L. H. Self-help groups: Types and psychological processes. *Journal of Applied Behavioral Science,* 1976, *12,* 310-322.

_____. Self-help groups viewed by mental health professionals: A survey and comments. *American Journal of Community Psychology,* 1978, *6,* 305-313.

Lieber, L. L., & Baker, J. M. Parents Anonymous and self-help treatment for child-abusing parents: A review and an evaluation. *Child Abuse and Neglect,* 1977, *1,* 133-148.

Lubchansky, I., Egri, G., & Stokes, J. Puerto Rican spiritualists view mental illness: The faith healer as a paraprofessional. *American Journal of Psychiatry,* 1970, *127,* 312-321.

McGuire, J., & Gottlieb, B. H. Social support groups among new parents: An experimental study in primary prevention. *Journal of Clinical Child Psychology,* 1979, *8,* 111-116.

Mowrer, O. H. Integrity Groups: Basic principles and procedures. *Counseling Psychologist*, 1972, *3*, 7-32.

———, & Vattano, A.J. Integrity groups: A context for growth in honesty, responsibility, and involvement. *Journal of Applied Behavioral Science*, 1976, *12*, 419-431.

President's Commission on Mental Health. *Task panel report: Community support systems*. February 1978. (NTIS No. PB-279801).

Prevention in Human Services, 1982, *1* (2).

Riessman, F. How does self-help work? *Social Policy*, 1976, *7*, 41-45.

Robinson, R., Demarche, D. F., & Wagle, M. K. *Community resources in mental health*. New York: Basic Books, 1960.

Rosenblatt, A., & Mayer, J. E. Help seeking for family problems: A survey of utilization and satisfaction. *American Journal of Psychiatry*, 1972, *128*, 126-130.

Rueveni, U. *Networking families in crisis*. New York: Human Sciences Press, 1979.

Ruiz, P., & Langrod, J. The role of folk healers in community mental health services. *Community Mental Health Journal*, 1976, *12*, 392-398.

Sarason, S. B. *The psychological sense of community: Prospects for a community psychology*. San Francisco: Jossey-Bass, 1974.

Sawin, M. M. *A background study paper on the theoretical assumptions of the family cluster model*. Unpublished manuscript, 1975. Available from Family Clustering, Inc., P.O. Box 18074, Rochester, N.Y.

Schwartz, M. D. Situation/transition groups: A conceptualization and review. *American Journal of Orthopsychiatry*, 1975, *45*, 744-755.

Silverman, P. R. The widow as a caregiver in a program of preventive intervention with other widows. *Mental Hygiene*, 1970, *54*, 540-547.

Social Policy, 1976, *1* (2).

Warren, D. I. *The neighborhood factor in problem coping, help seeking and social support: Research findings and suggested policy implications*. Paper presented at the meeting of the American Orthopsychiatric Association, San Francisco, March 1978.

———. Assessing community support systems in different types of neighborhoods. In J. Garbarino & H. Stocking (Eds.), *Protecting children from abuse and neglect*. San Francisco: Jossey-Bass, 1980.

Wechsler, H. The self-help organization in the mental health field: Recovery, Inc., a case study. *Journal of Nervous and Mental Disease*, 1960, *4*, 297-314.

Weiss, R. S. The contribution of an organization of single parents to the well-being of its members. *The Family Coordinator*, 1973, *22*, 321-326.

Zautra, A., & Simons, L. An assessment of a community's mental health needs. *American Journal of Community Psychology*, 1978, *6*, 351-362.

Chapter 13

CONSULTATION TO HUMAN SERVICE NETWORKS

Leonard D. Goodstein, Ph.D.

Human service organizations are those that offer services that either promote human welfare or reduce human misery. In most American communities of any size, the range and diversity of these organizations is enormous. The typical human service organization is characterized by an exclusive focus on a narrowly defined problem or on a restricted population. Some of these organizations serve only age-restricted groups, such as children or senior citizens; some serve only persons with certain kinds of problems, such as alcoholism or blindness; still others are concerned primarily with prevention rather than cure; yet another group of these agencies are concerned with rehabilitation of persons who previously were disabled. Not only have such a clarity of intent and a narrowness of focus been essential for the creation of the organization, but much of the continued community and fiscal support for such agencies may still depend upon exactly such a narrow mission. Neither human welfare nor human misery occurs in isolation, however, and the typical person needing help is frequently multiproblemed, with concerns that do not fit tidily into agency categories. Clients simply do not have problems that discriminate as neatly as agency mandates or criteria for service.

The specialization of agency services makes the services offered in a typical community a hodgepodge of overlap and underutilization, of redundancy and lack of coverage, of feast and famine. As Schulberg (1972) noted, a working mother may be able to readily obtain psychological consultation for her four-year-old child who is enrolled in a Head Start program but may be quite frustrated in obtaining the same help for her three-year-old who is too young for this program. Likewise, the parents of a developmentally disabled child may well have to negotiate individually with the departments of public health, mental health, and public welfare and the rehabilitation commission to make certain that the child receives all services and fiscal assistance to which that child is entitled. Even the most casual observer of our human service systems quickly recognizes that there is a need for creating systematic linkages that will bring together the several human service organizations in a genuinely effective system of service delivery.

As it now stands, however, most human service organizations operate as though their clients have a single, isolated problem that can be solved by that agency through its autonomous efforts. In most communities, human service systems are problem oriented rather than person oriented, and the responsibility for creating the necessary linkages to provide the range of services needed is all too often left to the client.

There are many exceptions to this observation, but the client is too frequently responsible for knowing that food stamps or whatever additional services are required can be obtained from another agency up the street or across town. The agency of initial contact may attempt to facilitate the link, but it would seem apparent that some degree of *bureaucratic competence* (Kahn, Katz, & Gutek, 1976) is necessary to negotiate this societal maze successfully. Yet, as Kahn, Katz, and Gutek showed, it is precisely the people who are most in need of such competence—the poor, the undereducated, and the minorities—who have the least of it. What is necessary is an organizational response that will take the place of such individual initiative.

Iscoe (1974), among others, advanced the concept of the *competent community* as one such societal alternative. The competent community is one that obtains, develops, and utilizes resources while having a primary focus on the full development of its members. Included among such resources would be the human service systems within that community. In such a competent community, the necessary linkages for providing a comprehensive system of human services would be indigenous to the structure of the several segments of the human service delivery system and of the community itself. Thus, rather than relying upon the bureaucratic competence of individuals to make the human service system operate effectively, the competent community would build the necessary linkages for comprehensive care into the fabric of the provider system and the community that supports such a system.

Any description of such a competent community at this time must be based upon hope and supposition, as no such community exists. But among the necessary characteristics of the human service delivery system in such a community would be a person orientation rather than the present problem orientation typical of our existing systems. It would not be necessary for an individual seeking help to deal with more than one care-giving institution even when there were multiple problems. Or if more than one agency or institution were involved, open and cordial communication between them and easily bridged boundaries would exist.

Community competence requires comprehensive services, integrated in a single agency or group of agencies, so that the entire range of human concerns that members of that community face can be confronted. The age- and problem-restricted care providers that typify our communities would be integrated into a unified, comprehensive system that could provide the linkages necessary for a total human service delivery system. Another characteristic of such a system would be coordination of all human services in order to make certain that all the services necessary for helping community members to cope with the complex and interrelated problems of our urban society would be available on a continuous basis. The care-giving system would be organized in such a way as to avoid unnecessary duplication of services while still providing those required. These services would be available in decentralized facilities in areas of high population density. Still a final characteristic of these services would be their proactive nature. Rather than continuing the passive stance typical of our current human care-giving agencies, in a competent community such organizations would be actively engaged in a variety of client-finding outreach activities working consistently toward removing the barriers to providing comprehensive human services.

HUMAN SERVICE NETWORKS

One step toward the development of the kind of human service delivery systems that we would expect to find in a competent community has been the development of human service networks. Human service networks are those systems concerned with establishment of linkages between existing and planned human service agencies. Rather than attempting to establish multiservice centers in which the constituent agencies would lose their identity and autonomy, the focus of the human service network is on facilitation of communication and referral, on reduction of interagency boundaries. Thus human service networks concentrate on issues of coordination and communication rather than upon integration and consolidation. Such an approach accepts the reality that, in most communities, it is not politically, financially, or practically feasible to integrate into a single, comprehensive facility all the services necessary in that community or neighborhood. The network concept accepts the reality of the existing tangled array of overlapping and competing agencies and attempts to operate such a chaotic system in a more rational, cooperative model.

These networks or consortia attempt to provide a coordination function, still typically centered around a fairly well defined problem area, such
as adolescents, runaways, child abuse, drug and alcohol abuse, or the
elderly. Although such networks are far from the comprehensive service
delivery system envisaged within the context of the competent community,
there is a conscious awareness that coordination, planning, and communication are necessary for effective service delivery. Such an awareness is
clearly the first step toward development of community competence, albeit
a small step.

Networks typically are created when one agency acknowledges that its
services are adversely affected by failure to arrange for other services that
can be provided only by another agency. The first agency calls a meeting of
the relevant community institutions, and there is some open discussion of
the need for coordination and communication, usually relying heavily upon
"horror stories," cases in which the failure of coordination had disastrous
outcomes. In one such case, a crisis counseling center that treated drug
abusers called a meeting to consider the total needs of the drug-abusing
client: psychological, medical, nutritional, vocational, and so on. The
meeting was precipitated by the problems the center encountered when a
client overdosed and nearly died before medical care could be obtained.

Following identification of the problem, there is then an attempt to
divide responsibilities according to expertise, available resources, and historical tradition. An agreement is reached to have an interface team or
coordinating council meet on some regular basis in order to explore how
well the coordination is working and to review cases in which problems
have developed. Typically considerable attention is paid to such matters as
rotating chairmanships, rotating meetings through the various participating agencies, and other structural elements that accentuate the fact that the
network is a congress of equals. In this case a drug abuse coordinating
council was created to provide an umbrella network for such services.
Although this council attempts to provide a communication channel among
the constituent agencies, it has little power to deal with problems except
through dialogue.

Human service networks are clearly on the increase. New federal and
state policies are forcing such collaboration in the interests of both greater
effectiveness and fiscal economy. The National Institute of Drug Abuse, for
example, is now developing the *single state agency* concept, whereby a
network will be established in each of the 50 states to coordinate the drug
abuse control programs, for all the reasons discussed earlier in this paper.
Federal funding will be solely to the single state agency, rather than to the
several community agencies as is now the case. From the federal
perspective, the single state agency concept is seen as a move toward local
control. From the perspective of the local community drug control

agencies, it is seen as a move from control at the more objective federal level to control at the more political state level. Nevertheless, the single state agency is but one of the many new mechanisms for establishing human service networks on a mandatory basis.

Since the network notion is aimed at increasing the overall quality of care provided to clients through the processes of communication, coordination, and collegiality, one must wonder why such networks did not develop earlier and more spontaneously and why there would ever be any problems in their operation. Some of the reasons lie in the nature of all human organizations, and others are a direct function of the special nature of human service systems. Using an open-systems approach (Katz & Kahn, 1978, discussed later in this chapter), we can see that all human organizations are concerned with boundary condition management (defining the organization's domain and maintaining the integrity of the domain) and negative entropy (preventing the system from running down, especially in the face of diminishing resources or competition for resources). Creation of a network accentuates concerns around both these issues which lead to competition, territoriality, suspiciousness, jealousy, and the other indexes of conflict that characterize most human service networks. These are the very issues that are most likely to lead to the need for consultation help.

SOME CHARACTERISTICS OF HUMAN SERVICE SYSTEMS

Some of the issues encountered in these networks stem from the intrinsic nature of human service systems. One such important characteristic is that the work done by such networks is not serially interdependent (Thompson, 1967). Such interdependence, which is typical of product manufacturing, requires that the output from one suborganization then be used as input for the other suborganization. In such interdependent systems, the success of the total organization is dependent upon the quality of the interdependence, and the failure of any part of a serially interdependent organization results in total organization failure.

In contrast with such natural and necessary interdependence, human service networks involve a forced or artificial interdependence. Dental care, for example, can be provided before, after, or independent of other services, such as speech therapy, counseling, special education, or food stamps. The output of any stage never becomes the *necessary* and exclusive input of the following stage. Thus the system or network is always a forced or artificial one.

Even more importantly, the various agencies involved in a network are never really dependent upon each other for either their own success or their continued survival. Each of the services offered by each of the agencies involved in a human service delivery network has its own market, its own budget, its own intrinsic worth, and its own system for social accountability. We may indeed recognize the need for treating the "whole client," but we, as a society, are quite willing to accept partial and incomplete services. Which service we prefer—mental health, child care, rehabilitation, depends upon our own peculiar values. Since the focus on treating the whole client tends to impinge upon the autonomy and separateness of the individual members of the network, the network never receives total allegiance from its members.

Another characteristic of human service systems is the way in which conflicts are managed. In these systems, conflicts are typically handled by "smoothing over," by denial, by compromising, by any means other than directly confronting the differences in an open manner. Openness about such differences permits them to become the focus of some conflict management processes. Instead, keeping conflict latent rather than manifest, that is, "sweeping differences under the rug," voicing harmony that is non-existent, pretending agreement when there is none, is typical of human service systems.

In my judgment, there are a number of possible explanations for this style of conflict management. One important consideration is that human service agencies are peopled by professionals who place high regard on interpersonal harmony and who regard conflict as destructive to both interpersonal relationships and the conduct of work. "Professional people just don't fight" is the way one social worker put it to me. But if such a credo means that real differences about agency policy and other important matters are never addressed, then a vital source of energy for growth and direction is lost.

A second reason for the development of these conflict-avoidant norms is inherent in the noninterdependent nature of human service delivery. By and large, what one worker does in providing service has very little impact on how the other workers in that agency provide services, just as what one agency does has little impact on what the other agencies do. Indeed, one of the important norms involved in being a professional is that each such person is a well-trained, competent individual who is best managed by allowing for autonomous exercise of the trained competence. Although one can advance other reasons to explain the strong conflict-avoidant norms of human service systems, it should be clear that there are substantial differences in conflict management between these systems and those in the profit-making sector. There are exceptions to this observation, but my experience has been that there is a great deal more open confrontation about differences in the private sector—in plant staff meetings, for example—than there ever is in the human service organizations with which I have worked. Efforts to open up the network, to facilitate people's "getting things off their chests,'' will have negative effects if there is not careful preparation for such openness and a carefully designed and widely accepted follow-up in which the hurts that often emerge from this kind of openness can be healed.

MODELS FOR CONSULTING WITH HUMAN SERVICE NETWORKS

Thus far attention has been devoted to an examination of human service networks, the agencies that are involved in such networks, and the ways they differ from other types of organizations. Although all three of the consultation models—educational, individual process, and system—are useful in working with human service networks, the preceding discussion clearly focuses on system issues, which suggests that a system model should be the primary model of intervention. One might hope that this is the case, but few organizations or networks have the necessary sophistication to recognize that their problems are systemic and to then seek a system-oriented consultation. Instead networks and organizations tend to respond to whatever issues are most disruptive and to seek help from either an educational or an individual-process model. Let us see how this happens.

Educational Model

In this case it is the client system that conceptualizes the problem as a lack of skill or knowledge. As the director of a mental health network might typically suggest: "Our problem is that our MBO [management-by-objectives] system just isn't working. Some of the agencies are OK and most aren't. Maybe the system isn't well designed and maybe it's just that our mental health professionals won't really engage in MBO, but what we need is an expert in MBO to review our system and then do some teaching of our managers about how to use MBO effectively." Similarly, a child care network director approached the consultant asking for a series of lectures on communication skills so that network personnel would have a better understanding of the nature of their communications—at least on some theoretical basis.

In both these cases, as in thousands more, the client system (or at least one powerful person in that system) has made a diagnostic judgment about the nature of the problem facing the system and has also prescribed an intervention strategy. Both these examples involve a self-diagnosis of lack of information and a decision to seek to remedy that information gap. Obviously in these cases, as is always true of intervention strategies, we have to start from where the client is, although there is usually a serious question about the adequacy of such a self-diagnosis.

Although some teaching about MBO or about communication skills may solve the client's problems, the identified concerns may be symptomatic of more basic and more pervasive problems. Rather than a problem in MBO, we may have a more general problem of inadequate leadership and a failure of upper management to define agency purpose. Rather than having a problem of a lack of communication skills, the child care staff may be suffering from problems of low cohesion, inadequate direction, and conflicting goal messages from the network director. Thus the central issue emerges: when to accept the client's diagnosis as adequate and when to question it.

First of all, it should be noted that any number of consultants have packaged programs for teaching performance appraisal, organizational behavior, communication skills, or whatever, and these consultants are ready and willing to provide these programs to the marketplace. Their general approach is a commercial one. They describe their programs fairly and sell these programs to whomever is willing to buy them. If there is any caution, it clearly is caveat emptor. I am not suggesting any dishonesty or immorality in such an approach; it simply differs from that espoused by a professional model of consultation. In such a model, the client and the consultant jointly agree to review the symptoms or the causes for concern, to consider the possible reasons for these symptoms, to develop a series of potential intervention strategies, to consider the potential cost-benefit consequences of these strategies, and then to go ahead with a mutually agreed upon course of action. Not all programs of intervention—medical, legal, educational, or psychological—are carried out according to this formula, but it does represent the best professional model. The true professional does not insist that "the doctor knows best," but neither is there a willingness to agree that "the consumer is always right." The commercial model of consultation does assume the latter, a value very much in keeping with the marketplace orientation followed by all too many consultants.

Second, if one does follow the professional model, how can one proceed? The consultant may agree that an educational intervention is one possible strategy and that he or she can provide such an intervention but, at the same time, begins to question the client's data base and the processes by which the client decided to use a particular intervention strategy. In other words, the consultant who agrees with the client's presentation of the problem as one way of considering the situation may begin to use his or her awareness of system issues to open up an additional series of alternatives. Although it may be that, in the final analysis, the client was right and some educational program is useful as a first step, the consultant has broadened the client's understanding of the system, of how to go about diagnosing problems in the system, and of what possible interventions may follow from a variety of diagnoses.

There are many examples of educational interventions that followed from such a diagnosis. A major American airline was experiencing severe problems with its ground counter personnel, who had become abusive to passengers when flights were delayed or cancelled. The consultants who were called in to help solve the problem interviewed a large number of these agents and found that the passengers seemed to them to behave "childishly" when their flights were not on time. In observing the agents' response to this behavior, the consultants saw that the agents then responded "parentally." This observation suggested that some kind of training in transactional analysis might help the agents understand the dynamics of their own behavior and change it accordingly. A large-scale transactional analysis training program was initiated, with a highly beneficial result in terms of reduced passenger complaints, reduced absenteeism, and reduced turnover on the part of agents. Clearly an educational model is useful in consulting with human service systems, but consultants need to be wary about uncritically accepting the client's stated needs or desires for particular training programs or training packages.

Individual-Process Model

The individual-process model is probably the least widely used model in working with human service networks, indeed, with any organizations. Not that individual processes are not operating in organizations, but rather conceptualization and intervention are typically at a group or system level. Attitudes are always carried on the individual level, but when they are widely shared within an ongoing group or organization, they become part of the psychological characteristics of that organization, part of its norms and values. Indeed, the process of socialization into an organization (Katz and Kahn, 1978) attempts to make certain that all new members of the organization "buy into" these norms and values. One of the problems typically experienced by former mental health practitioners who become organizational consultants is to attribute too much causality to the attitudes and behavior of single individuals and not to pay enough attention to the pervasive organizational climate that affects everyone who works in that setting.

Nevertheless, at times an individual-process model, with its attention to mental health-related problems, is necessary in organizational consultation. It does happen that a single individual's behavior can have strong negative effects on an organization, especially if that person is in a position of power or influence. In one such case involving a network providing comprehensive services for the elderly, very little work was getting done and a high level of frustration was being reported by many of the staff workers. All this led to a request for consultation help. The consultant quickly determined that one supervisor, perplexed and bewildered by the pressure for integration of services and open communication in the new network, simply had become immobilized and had retreated into a psychotic-like withdrawal accompanied by a good bit of paranoid ideation.

Personal concern for the individual and an unwillingness to confront the problem had snowballed, and no one either in the individual's unit or in the network was willing to take the necessary steps to exit the individual on even a temporary basis. The consultant quickly recognized the nature of the person's emotional state and helped arrange a leave of absence and a referral to a competent mental health practitioner. Although the consultant himself chose not to deal with problems posed by this individual as they affected the network, it was his awareness of and willingness to address these issues that is characteristic of the individual-process model. Whether or not the organizational consultant chooses to use the individual-processes model, it is clear that there needs to be continuous awareness of how the personal attitudes, motivations, intrapsychic conflicts, and emotional disturbances of individuals can affect organizational and system functioning.

System Model

Since networks are systems, it should not be surprising that a system model for consultation has the widest utility. Although the entry of consultants into human service networks is very often based upon an educational model, even utilization of the educational model needs to be understood in system terms. Introducing a token economy program, for example, in a rehabilitation network can be done through an educational model, but if the networkwide implications of adopting such a model are not worked through, the program is unlikely to be successful. Introducing such a program is certain to involve such issues as which clients are entered in the program, how they are to be moved into and out of the program, and who is to manage the program. The effects of introducing any substantial change in a network will ripple through the network and have profound, long-term implications. Most programmatic changes in organizations that fail do so because of failure of the persons responsible for the innovation to conceptualize the organization in system terms and plan accordingly. Of special concern is the differential commitment to the innovation in the several constituent agencies.

When most of us are asked to describe an organization with which we are familiar, we tend to draw the organization chart, with its hierarchically arranged boxes, in order to explain how things are organized. Such a static model of an organization is inadequate to describe the important psychological characteristics of any organization, its patterns of communication, power, support, and influence. An open-system model of organizational life (Katz & Kahn, 1978) is a far more adequate model since it is concerned with the elements of the system, the structure of the system, the inter-dependency of elements of the system, and the way the system is embedded in the environment.

Open-system theory conceptualizes organizations as patterns of recurrent activities in which energy (information, personnel, raw materials) is imported into the system and transformed in some fashion or another, and the resulting product (or service in the case of human service networks) is exported back into the environment. In contrast with the closed-system notions that stem from classical Newtonian physics, open systems maintain themselves through a constant interchange with the host environments, and thus there is a continuous exchange of energy between the system and its environment. The analog of the open-system model is the living cell, not a static hydraulic system.

Thus an open system involves a recurring cycle of input, transformation, and output. Both the input and output characteristics of the open system keep the system in constant commerce with the environment, and the transformation process is contained within the system. An effective open system requires a balance between the three stages of the cycle, with the input taking into account both environmental demands and the capacity of the transformation cycle and the transformation process absorbing the flow from the input and moving to the output stage. Levinson and Astrachan (1976) provided an excellent example of how such an open-system model helps explain the role of the intake staff in a community mental health program and the problems such a staff encounters in regulating the organization's boundary conditions. The intake staff held the important and primary responsibility ''of regulating the patient-input boundary so as to import an appropriate patient population at a manageable rate'' (p. 22). As Levinson and Astrachan went on to point out, when the intake staff takes in more patients than the transformation (or treatment) system can handle, the overflow patients are neglected, transferred or referred elsewhere, or discharged early through the ''revolving door.'' By contrast, the intake staff might be highly selective, admitting only a special group of ''suitable'' patients and turning large numbers away. This method might meet the treatment staff's criteria of suitability, but the failure to meet environmental needs leads to a loss of support from the surrounding community. Thus the task of the intake staff is to manage a delicate balance between demand and capability, between environmental need and internal resources, or it will lose credibility in managing its interface between the organization and its environment. The problem of managing boundary conditions in a network is even more difficult, as there is much more uncertainty about the nature of the task assumed by the network and there also is a larger environment involved—a more diffuse and ambiguous constituency.

This brief example should give the reader some inkling of the utility of open-system models in understanding organizational life. The organizational consultant who can operate from this model can begin to understand some of the intrinsic issues that will continuously emerge in organizations as input, transformation, and output are interminably repeated. Such a consultant will understand that, in the example, the problems involved in the role of the intake staff are never solvable in any final sense, but rather there is a dynamic tension that must always exist in those segments of the organization responsible for boundary condition management as they attempt to balance the conflicting interests of the system and the environment. The solution that worked today will almost certainly not work tomorrow. False expectations about final solutions are important factors in producing ''burnout'' in such intake staffs.

An Operational Model

Open-system theory provides an overview and a theoretical structure through which a system-oriented consultant can function in working with networks, but it does not provide much in the way of an operational guide for consultation. One such operational guide is found in the work of Weisbord (1978), whose model of organizational diagnosis and consultation is based upon open-system theory and is one that works quite well with networks.

Weisbord provided a semistandardized series of questions, rating forms, and areas of inquiry that focus the attention of the consultant on six interrelated organizational processes that are involved in organizational networks and that need to be understood by consultants and their clients. The six processes are (1) purpose, (2) structure, (3) relationships, (4) rewards, (5) leadership, and (6) helpful mechanisms.

The *purposes* or goals of the network involve both the clarity of these goals and the degree of commitment to the goals by its members. Obviously the former is necessary for the latter. One of the most important characteristics of human service networks is low goal clarity, suggesting that one of the problems system-oriented consultants will encounter most often is the need for increasing goal clarity. In such networks there will be confusion over how the network developed, why it is needed, how it should function, and what its future directions should be. The strong norms of conflict avoidance make uncovering these issues difficult. The consultant needs to help members of the network admit and accept differences about goals, differences that may have remained latent over time. This is not a simple task, and it is one that requires time and energy for both client and consultant.

Taber, Walsh, and Cooke (1979) reported on their problems in consulting to a community services council that emerged in response to a crisis situation: the closing down of a plant that was a major employer in the community. They noted that their major efforts were directed at helping this network and its constituent agencies develop a *domain consensus,* that is, a clarity of goal or purpose. Indeed, so threatened were some institutions by the establishment of the network that they refused even to participate in the early meetings, at which goal setting was the only order of business. Establishment of goal clarity is clearly no simple matter.

An analysis of *structure* involves both the formal organization chart and, even more important, the informal social structure that helps work get done (or hinders it). One important consideration in working with networks is that the necessary interdependency between units is typically lower than the interdependency within units of the network. The organizational consultant working with a network needs to consider how much teamwork between units of the network is really necessary for task accomplishment and to strive for such teamwork when necessary. Since many consultants operating in human services have a strong value commitment to teamwork, even when it is not necessary for task performance, such a warning is necessary.

Occasionally, however, the structural elements of the client system require attention, especially in newly established networks. In one such case, I was asked to help identify and solve the organizational problems experienced by a job-training network (Goodstein, 1972). The network involved two bureaucracies, one for state rehabilitation workers and the other for municipal school district teachers. Communication between a counselor and a teacher working on the same case could occur only on a formal basis, by sending a memo up the hierarchy, across at the level of the codirectors, and then down, a process that could take a week. The two workers were more than a little frustrated by the process, and most of the agency's clients lost interest before any important decision could be made. One important intervention was the consultant's focusing on this structural problem and pushing the network to consider how it could be reduced or eliminated.

The *relationships* that may be involved in a network include the interpersonal, the intergroup, and the interactive ones between the employees and the technology. Since there is typically little technology involved in human service systems, this last kind of interaction tends to have little importance there. As we noted earlier, there is a strong norm in human service systems that interpersonal and intergroup conflict, especially the former, is "unprofessional" and that human service workers, especially those professionally trained, need to get along. The impact of this norm is to sweep conflict "under the rug" and to pretend agreement that does not exist. Such a failure to confront differences might be assumed to have a disastrous effect upon human service organizations, but this is not the case.

The low interdependence in such organizations permits the typical conflict avoidance to work reasonably well, except when real collaboration is necessary, as in long-range planning. Indeed, the inability of these systems to accept differences among members of the organization may be seen as critical in reducing their effectiveness and provides another entry point for the system-oriented consultant.

Organizational *rewards* include both formal rewards, such as raises, promotions, bonuses, and the like, and the more informal, personal rewards and support that a supervisor can give for work well done. In most human service networks, supervisors and managers tend to focus their attention on the former and overlook the latter. The former, however, are difficult to use because of the way such rewards are managed bureaucratically, aside from the question about how well such rewards motivate people in any event. In working with these systems, consultants need to be aware of the limitations that typically exist in using the formal reward structure and instead concentrate upon helping the system use the informal, psychological rewards more effectively.

The role of *leadership* in an organization is to keep the other elements of the system in balance and to constantly monitor the functioning of the system. In most human service systems, the task of leadership is poorly understood and there is very little legitimization of a leadership function. The assumption all too often is that the workers are highly trained and competent professionals and the system runs itself. In our example of the job-retraining center, the roles of the two codirectors were developed to assure parity of power rather than to provide effective leadership. Each of the incumbents spent most of his time blocking or thwarting any attempts by the other to move the network off dead center. One need that the consultant thus may encounter frequently is for a clearer understanding of the role of an organizational leader and the way that role can be adequately filled. Here there may be a need for both a theory-based input using an educational model and a system-based intervention that focuses on the destructive consequences of the failure to provide leadership in this network.

The *helpful mechanisms*, such as budgeting, management information systems, and evaluation research, plus the way in which such systems are used, are the last of Weisbord's six processes. Unfortunately, all too often these systems are absent, poorly implemented, or abused in human service networks. The typical budgeting procedures in human service networks require that future budgets be pegged at previous levels of client services, using a rather narrow definition of client service. Such a budgeting process makes innovation and change very difficult and tends to reduce the interest of the network in developing cost-effectiveness. When consultants are brought into such networks, these consultants need to be aware that such helpful mechanisms must be integrated into an overall system approach to the agency and that there will be strong resistance to such budgeting processes through the organization.

SUMMARY AND CONCLUSIONS

Human service systems touch all our lives as citizens and consumers. Further, those of us who are mental health professionals spend most of our lives working in such systems. The need to have such systems operate both effectively and humanely should be immediately obvious to even the most casual observer.

For those who are interested in consulting with human service systems, either as external to the system or as internal change agents, I have attempted to delineate some of the specific characteristics of these systems that need to be involved. I have presented a brief overview of Weisbord's model of understanding organizations as one system-oriented model for working with human service networks, and I have pointed out how the educational and individual-processes models complement the system model. Clearly there is much that could be added. There are fairly well developed and tested strategies (see Goodstein, 1978, for a further discussion of these) for consulting with human service systems. Such a system approach can readily be expanded to conceptualize problems of social service networks. Such networks are characterized as having difficulty in establishing any domain consensus, as having low interdependence, and as being prone to covert conflict over issues of territoriality. Both those who would work as consultants in social service networks and those who would be consumers of such help need to be adequately informed about the research and theory that is now available.

REFERENCES

Goodstein, L. D. Organizational development as a model for community consultation. *Hospital & Community Psychiatry,* 1972, *23,* 165-168.
_____. *Consulting with human service systems.* Reading, Mass.: Addison-Wesley, 1978.
_____ & Boyer, R. K. Crisis intervention in a municipal agency: A conceptual case history. *Journal of Applied Behavioral Science,* 1972, *8,* 318-340.
Iscoe, I. Community psychology and the competent community. *American Psychologist,* 1974, *29,* 607-613.

Kahn, R. L., Katz, D., & Gutek, B. Bureaucratic encounters—An evaluation of government services. *Journal of Applied Behavioral Science,* 1976, *12,* 178-198.

Katz, D., & Kahn, R. L. *Social psychology of organization* (2nd ed.). New York: Wiley, 1978.

Levinson, D., & Astrachan, B. Entry into the mental health center: A problem in organizational boundary regulation. In E. J. Miller (Ed.), *Task and organization.* London: Wiley, 1976.

Schulberg, H. C. Challenge of human service programs for psychologists. *American Psychologist,* 1972, *27,* 566-573.

Taber, T. D., Walsh, J. T., & Cooke, R. A. Developing a community-based program for reducing the social impact of a plant closing. *Journal of Applied Behavioral Science,* 1979, *15.*

Thompson, J. D. *Organizations in action.* New York: McGraw-Hill, 1967.

Weisbord, M. *Organizational diagnosis.* Reading, Mass.: Addison-Wesley, 1978.

Chapter 14

FUTURE DIRECTIONS FOR CONSULTATION BY MENTAL HEALTH SYSTEMS

Donald C. Klein, Ph.D.

In theory, the mental health field upholds some of our civilization's highest values. Going far beyond provision of treatment and rehabilitation, its mandate encompasses maintenance of entire populations' mental health. Mental health systems are supposed by some to be focusing attention on the welfare of groups deemed to be at high risk of manifesting "needless psychopathology" (Goldston, 1977). To carry out this mandate, they of course would need to involve themselves with the many formal and informal facets of communities that are presumed to have an impact on the emotional well-being of large numbers of people.

The track record of the mental health movement falls far short of the movement's far-ranging potential. Federally funded community mental health programs have spent, on the average, 95 percent of their time on treatment and rehabilitation and only 5 percent on those consultation and education activities that are essential if the larger mandate is to be honored. The mental health enterprise, as it has evolved to this point, works diligently to help selected individuals concentrate on the nature of their problems and ways to overcome them; it allows the steady supply of psychopathology to remain unchecked. In effect, it functions so as to ensure that the supply of individuals seeking treatment as patients of the mental health system will remain virtually constant and certainly unending.

There is some reason to believe that the creation of mental health treatment facilities can be counterproductive for the emotional well-being of the community at large, at least over the long run. The reasoning behind this supposition—which, it must be acknowledged, has never been seriously studied and documented—is that clergy, educators, and other community care-takers, when they refer people to mental health specialists, tend to remove themselves from assuming primary responsibility for the emotional well-being of their clientele. Thus as a mental health center gains visibility and enjoys increased community confidence, people who heretofore would have taken their emotional concerns to friends, neighbors, and professional care givers are channeled instead to mental health specialists. In the process, the natural care-taking functions of the community are weakened, if not altogether supplanted.[1]

The counterproductivity of the present state of affairs was reflected in the report of the President's Commission on Mental Health (*Report to the President*, 1978). The report placed renewed emphasis on prevention and called for more flexible deployment of resources via mental health *systems* rather than sole reliance on bureaucratically structured mental health *centers*. The impetus for redeployment comes from a variety of sources. These include a growing band of mental health workers themselves. They are aware of a growing body of research pointing to modest successes for preventive programs with specific target populations and for general efforts to promote more effective problem solving and coping among children. In the light of these data, they believe it is important to develop ways to deploy such programs and to improve them on a populationwide basis. The pioneer work of Hans Selye and others who recognize the unitary nature of the organism in response to environmental stressors has engendered an increasingly holistic view of the task of health maintenance. This view, in turn, has led to increasingly widespread attempts to institutionalize health maintenance models integrating mind, body, and spirit in their applications.

CONSULTATION AS A CENTRAL STRATEGY

I foresee that such developments will have far-reaching effects on the use of consultation by mental health centers. Until now mental health consultation has tended to be an ancillary function performed as a supplement to clinical services; in the future it will become an increasingly central strategy as mental health systems take seriously their responsibility to disseminate knowledge and promote social changes that will be in the interest of disease prevention and enhancement of emotional well-being within entire populations.

As I see it, if mental health consultation becomes part of a central strategy for mental health, as I think it will, the purposes to which it will be put probably will include the following:

1. Promoting healthy growth and development among those whose lives have not yet been scarred by psychopathology

2. Multiplying and strengthening helping services, outside the mental health center, available to those already in need of emotional reeducation and rehabilitation

3. Fostering the best possible use of patient care services offered by mental health agencies by ensuring earliest possible case finding and suitable referral of those in need

4. Helping establish interpersonal and institutional supports for those at risk of emotional disorder at various points in the life cycle and when faced with unexpected life challenges

5. In its fullest realization, allying the mental health field with those in the position to create *competent communities,* by which I mean communities that provide physical and psychological security for all citizens, that foster effective coping and problem solving, and that enable all persons to enjoy lives filled with significance, in their eyes and those of others (Klein, 1968).

NEEDED STRUCTURAL CHANGES

There are three structural and technical considerations with which mental health planners and policymakers must grapple as they move toward fuller realization of the aforementioned potentials.

First, consultation typically is embedded in a treatment-oriented system designed to respond to immediate, day-by-day service demands of troubled people. The administrative and programmatic design of the typical mental health center is far more responsive to processing of patients from intake through disposition to the point of discharge than it is geared to the temporal, managerial, and resource requirements of so-called indirect services. Indeed, as Swift emphasized,[2] the very distinction of "direct" clinical and "indirect" community services reflects a basic mind set wherein the principal responsibility of the mental health system is to assist with emotional distress rather than forestall it. In order for consultation to be fully utilized, it must enter into equal status with other functions. To do so, the mind set, programmatic priorities, and ethical considerations of the mental health system must also be altered. I expect there will be growing recognition that it makes no more sense for preventively oriented programs in mental health to be tied to treatment-oriented institutions than it would for a community's public health department to be subsumed under its general hospital's administration.

The natural home of a preventively oriented mental health effort is a population-oriented setting committed to the public's health, the latter being broadly defined to include the general well-being of all individuals in a target area. This idea is neither original nor new. It permeated the thinking of some of the pioneers in community-based mental health programming. Similarly, some of the most imaginative broad-gauge general health promotion programs (e.g., the Peckham experiment in England, reported by Farber, 1976, and Pearse & Crocker, 1943) have institutionally encompassed a concern for the whole person, body as well as mind. Recent innovations in so-called holistic health may reflect a resurgence of this historic emphasis in public health. It should be abundantly clear that the mind-body integration works both ways. Not only does mind affect body; it is equally apparent that care of the body (as, for example, via exercise and proper nutrition) is reflected in an elevation of the spirit and a general increase in emotional well-being. Therefore I look forward to the time when mental health consultation, no longer a separate enterprise, has become but one aspect of an integrative orientation for health and general well-being.

Second, deployment of mental health services within delimited catchment areas provides another structural barrier to the most expeditious deployment of consultation, to at least two groups: (1) large agencies whose boundaries extend beyond the catchment areas; (2) certain constellations of care-taking resources located without regard to catchment area boundaries. Most major human service systems (e.g., schools, courts, public and private recreation programs) are administered on a citywide basis or via sections within a metropolitan area. Moreover, many of them are profoundly affected by significant influences and inputs from state or national funding sources and policymakers. The future deployment of mental health consultation will need to reflect such geographical considerations. Various possibilities are already being explored, among them consortia of mental health centers serving a metropolitan area, which can contract with major care-taking agencies such as the schools; and separately financed and administered consultation and education programs, which may sponsor projects and undertake contracts beyond specific catchments.

As these structural considerations are taken into account, I believe consultative work will become better able to encompass improvement of major systems of our communities, both internally and with respect to how well the systems collaborate in the interests of clients. Our mental health efforts will become more seriously engaged in efforts to transform the educational and other human service functions of our society in the interests of reducing the steady stream of psychiatric casualties. Such an enlargement of vision does not preclude a continuation of case-oriented mental health consultation. Rather it presages an extension of mental health consultants' competence to include skills that at present are to be found primarily among consultants in organizational development and applied behavioral scientists, who attempt to integrate personal development and systemic effectiveness.

The preponderance of evidence from these sources supports the thesis that involvement of organization members in systemic decision making has a favorable impact on the well-being of both systems and their personnel (Hall, 1976). Also available are a range of reasonably well evaluated consultative approaches, a substantial knowledge base, and a value orientation that seems entirely suitable for the mental health field. By adapting approaches from the applied behavioral sciences, mental health consultants will be in a position to contribute to the cultivation of more effective formal and informal community support systems.

Third, the effectiveness of current efforts in mental health consultation is limited by inability to monitor trends and identify priority needs within populations. The need has long been recognized for ongoing epidemiologic systems to keep track of the distribution and rates of occurrence of psychopathology on a communitywide basis. Early efforts, for example, in Wellesley (Klein & Lindemann, 1964), Nova Scotia (Leighton, 1956), and New York City (Srole, Langer, Michael, Opler, & Rennie, 1962), demonstrated both the many difficulties involved and the potential guidance such efforts afford. The aim must be to focus consultation and other interventions on behalf of those at greatest risk. Despite the considerable technical, attitudinal, and values considerations that remain, I am still convinced that an epidemiologic basis for consultation and other mental health services will ultimately be achieved without sacrificing civil liberties or the right to personal privacy. Case-by-case accounting systems are by no means the only available approach. Surveys of physical and emotional well-being, use of care takers as informal observers, and localized in-community application of social indicator methods are additional options that await refinement.

CHANGING CONSULTANTS' MIND SET

Beyond the aforementioned structural and technologic changes, there are two fundamental changes needed in the mind set of the mental health consultant that I believe are forthcoming. The first involves the shift from a clinical case-oriented model to one that is concerned with the ecology of systems and events. An ecological orientation already forms the undergirding for much of community psychology theory and training (Iscoe, Bloom, & Spielberger, 1977) and is finding its way into mental health practice via such means as therapeutic communities and family therapy. An ecological orientation, as has been emphasized elsewhere (e.g., Bateson, 1975; Kelly, 1968), involves a fundamental shift in consciousness and in our understanding of how change occurs.

Following the ecological model, we know that any phenomenon is held in place by a complex array of factors or forces, none of which can be considered either the ''cause'' or the ''effect'' of behavior that concerns us. The model challenges the illusory dichotomies of cause-effect, right-wrong, villain-victim that have dominated the consensual illusions of Western society for thousands of years. Applying the ecological orientation to current shifts in patterns of marriage and divorce, for example, it is possible to see that such major changes are associated in a complex fashion with the system of interstate highways that has been stimulated by and, in turn, has accelerated individual and family mobility. There is not a unidirectional causal influence in the interaction among these and associated sociocultural and technologic factors. Indeed, given the combined technologies of mass transportation and communication, the associated mobility that both fosters and results from such technologies, and their impact on family life, increased divorce rates are inevitable concomitants.

With an ecological orientation, mental health consultation becomes a process whereby the mental health system deliberately becomes part of a community's ecology with the intention of facilitating a milieu that promotes emotional well-being. Informed by a vision of such a community, the consultant engages with consultee systems in the effort to create alterations of the ecological field. To do so, it is important to get to know the ecology of the community, to understand the forces holding it in place, and to devise those interventions that, with the least possible effort, may facilitate a transformation of circumstances. I look forward to the time when the consciousness of mental health consultants will enable them to forego the simpler cause-effect model, thereby opening up myriad possibilities for innovative interventions.

Awareness of the importance of the ecological orientation presages even more far-reaching reorientations of thinking and practice in mental health. We stand on the threshhold of a major revolution in our understanding of human behavior, one that will be even more transforming in its social implications than the ones that removed chains from mental patients or made *the unconscious* a byword in our time. The antecedents of the projected revolution are diverse. They include the major technological shifts affecting mobility and communication which are associated with increased instability of beliefs and cultural patterns. They are also to be found in several major discoveries and formulations of psychology and social sciences that have materially affected everyday conceptions of personal and social reality. They began with the psychodynamic formulations of the early 1900s, which proposed that it is possible to bring potentially destructive instinctual forces under the conscious control of the ego. Almost simultaneously, there arose the revolutionary explorations of human learning that engendered the realization that behavior followed certains laws and could, under proper circumstances, be deliberately shaped and modified. By midcentury the cybernetic revolution was under way. Its emphasis on the potency of human systems and the ubiquity of the feedback principle opened the doors to an avalanche of knowledge and technology having to do with planned change in interpersonal, group, and organizational behavior. The cybernetic revolution has enabled large numbers of people to learn how to participate with others at a heretofore unheard of level of interpersonal awareness. It has spawned a new training and consultation industry having to do with organizational development, integration of concerns for person and task, and facilitation of planned change in response to the vision of improved organizational and community functioning. Then hard on the heels of the cybernetic revolution came the dissemination of the concept of perceptual relativity, perhaps most clearly exemplified by the gestalt therapy movement, which undertook to enable people to claim their own feelings and acknowledge responsibility for their own reactions.

The most recent antecedents are to be found in our rediscovery of the phenomenon of transpersonal reality based on acknowledgment of oneness with a universal consciousness of which every living being is a part. Previously reserved for seemingly esoteric Eastern disciplines, transpersonal reality has attracted the attention of serious students and practitioners in mental health. Its recent manifestations include a growing recourse to meditation and relaxation techniques for purposes of treatment and prevention and the integration of mind, body, and spirit within the growing "holistic" health movement.

What is emerging is an exciting positive vision of a world that tunes into a higher level of consciousness. The vision acknowledges that the sensory world in which we find ourselves is essentially a creation of our minds. At the heart of the dawning consciousness is the realization that individuals do not need to invest their sense of self-worth in defending their views of reality against their own or others' disconfirming experiences or perceptions. Individuals are capable of expressing more positively directed energy and of finding joyful feelings in their experience of consciousness. Under such circumstances it is possible to envision an almost unlimited potential for competent, caring communities of people for whom joy and zest for living would constitute fundamental aspects of their personal lives and their relations with one another. My own experience tells me that, having once accepted the fundamental fact of the mind-as-creator-of-reality, one enters a state of being in which one experiences genuine unconditional positive regard not only for clients (as suggested by Carl Rogers) but also for oneself and indeed for all events impinging on one's life.

The implications for mental health consultation should be far reaching. Reducing or eliminating misconceptions of belief and self-importance, mental health consultation will be able to turn its attention to helping consultees free themselves and their institutions from unnecessary attachment to their conceptions and beliefs about what is real and right. Key care-taking groups will discover ways to foster optimal growth and development among those in their care, to reduce dysfunctional discontinuities in the life cycle, to build firm supports at points of challenge and transition, and to help their clients play the game of life more knowingly and with more zest. The effects would be to reduce the pervasive social paranoia occasioned by personal and social insecurity and to build social institutions that functioned as if people mattered.

I expect that mental health consultants will become less involved in focusing on problems and increasingly predisposed to exploring with their consultees the possibilities for joyful coping. Their efforts will become increasingly suffused with an educational rather than a clinical orientation. In effect, they will be conveying a fundamental approach to healthy growth and development based on raised consciousness and a new appreciation of the integrity of mind, body, and matters of the spirit.

At the outset of this chapter, I was setting myself the delightful challenge of shaping visions as well as predicting future directions. Each reader will, of course, make the final decision about his or her future. I am satisfied that at the core of everyone's consciousness is the knowledge that what I have described alludes to a kernel of truth, however much it may have been distorted by the limitations of words and subtle distortions of my own beliefs and preconceptions.

NOTES

1. This process could be envisioned as going on virtually indefinitely. No mental health center has yet plumbed the depths of the available pool of potential patients. If one accepts the thesis that emotional problems are as prevalent as the common cold, that pool is inexhaustible, embracing as it may virtually all of a community's inhabitants one or more times in their lives.

2. Swift, C. Personal communication. 1980.

REFERENCES

Bateson, G. *Steps to an ecology of mind.* New York: Ballantine Books, 1975.

Farber, A. The Peckham experiment revisited: Cultivating health. *Health and Social Work,* 1976, *1*(3), 27-38.

Goldston, S. An overview of primary prevention programming. In D. Klein & S. Goldston (Eds.), *Primary prevention: An idea whose time has come* (DHEW Pub. [ADM] 77-447.). Washington, D.C., 1977.

Hall, J. To achieve or not: The manager's choice. *California Management Review,* 1976, *18,* 5-18.

Iscoe, I., Bloom, B., & Spielberger, C. (Eds.). *Community psychology in transition.* New York: Wiley, 1977.

Kelly, J. Toward an ecological conception of preventive interventions. In J. W. Carter (Ed.), *Research contributions from psychology to community mental health.* New York: Behavioral Publications, 1968.

Klein, D. *Community dynamics and mental health.* New York: Wiley, 1968.

_____. & Lindemann, E. Approaches to pre-school screening. *Journal of School Health,* 1964, *34,* 365-373.

Leighton, D. The distribution of psychiatric symptoms in a small town. *American Journal of Psychiatry,* 1956, *112,* 716-723.

Pearse, I., & Crocker, L. *The Peckham experiment.* London: Allen and Unwin, 1943.

Report to the President from the President's Commission on Mental Health. Washington, D.C.: U.S. Government Printing Office, 1978.

Srole, L., Langer, T. S., Michael, S. T., Opler, M. K., & Rennie, T. A. C. *Mental health in the metropolis.* New York: McGraw-Hill, 1962.

Part V

CONCLUSIONS

Chapter 15

IN CONCLUSION
The Past, Present, and Future in
Consultation

Noel A. Mazade, Ph.D.

This chapter will seek to provide an overview of several issues highlighted throughout this publication that are related to various aspects of consultation theory and practice. The previous authors have individually and collectively provided a variety of viewpoints regarding the status of consultation in the mental health field and its contribution as a helping process, as an agent of social change, and a promising tool for influencing the overall prevalence of mental disorder in the community.[1]

In illustrating their various individual ideas, the authors have presented a number of explicit and implicit aspects of general consultation practice independent of specific consultation "type" (i.e., case, program, community, etc.). This final chapter will discuss the generic issues in an effort to both summarize the state of the art and raise several methodological and theoretical considerations for the future.

THE FIELD AND DEFINITION OF CONSULTATION

As documented by several authors, the mental health enterprise embraced consultation as a methodology following Caplan's and others' pioneering efforts, first, to "discover" the existence of consultation as a technique worth utilizing, and second, to differentiate its various forms and functions. Since this early work, much effort has been directed toward both refining consultation practice and institutionalizing it within the skill repertoire of the fields of community mental health and community psychology.

As a basic and legislatively required service within federally funded community mental health centers, consultation (and education) moved from a concept to a functioning program entity. As such, new considerations arose including (but not limited to) issues of funding, development of a "market," community acceptance, personnel, training of consultant staff, and evaluation. Likewise, within the field of community psychology, these and other issues have assumed paramount importance since consultation methods constitute key implementation strategies for fulfilling the goals espoused by this emerging discipline.

Given the dependence between successful practice and the availability of fiscal and human resources, the consultation practice field can no longer be considered only within the confines of discussion related to methodology or consultation's potential for ultimately increasing the level of mental health. Rather, as noted by Bowen and Collett (1978), the consultation field must be considered a "growth industry, with all the problems and opportunities inherent in growth" (p. 476). As society attempts to find more effective and efficient methods for accomplishing goals, public- and private-sector organizations, groups, and individuals will call upon consultants of all types for assistance. When perceived from a system perspective, consultation practice must be viewed by all parties within and without the mental health system in relation to the tension and pressures created when any expenditure of funds and resources is compared with the ultimate efficacy of results achieved. In considering those pressures specifically in relation to management consultation, Bowen and Collett (1978) noted that "the consequences such pressures hold in the competition for capable management consultants on one hand and the development of quality consultant resources on the other pose substantial public interest problems" (p. 476).

These public interest considerations are by no means insignificant, either within or without the mental health field. From the early days of the independent child guidance movement (when psychiatrists provided *case consults* to other professionals) to the current period (in which 2 percent of all federally funded grant expenditures for community mental health centers is mandated for technical assistance, including consultation), the field of mental health has expended millions of dollars and logged innumerable episodes of consultation. In the nonpublic sector, thousands of business enterprises are devoted to the function of consultation. Pattenaude (1979) noted an early Cornell University study that forecast that, by the end of the 1970s, nearly 8,000 firms—not included small, informal firms or individuals in private consultation practice—would be involved in consulting activities. As evidence of this development, Sterling (1977) indicated that, in 1976 alone, the federal government let $110 billion in contracts to nonfederal agencies of which $60 billion went to contracting units in the private sector.

Thus, in viewing this nationally emerging proprietary enterprise, public mental health consultants must consider the ultimate probability of their continued existence in a less parochial and holistic framework. As a "public interest" enterprise, the mental health consultation field will be increasingly compelled to establish its legitimacy as a viable and useful product, to assess its potential and ability to compete with the existing and rapidly expanding private firms specializing in consultation, and to develop strategies to train competent and credible consultants who can function effectively in a variety of contexts. At this writing, such issues are assuming even more immediate relevance since much of the governmental funding that has supported consultation practice through grants to community mental health centers, universities, and other agencies and institutions has begun to evaporate. Having few fixed and/or visible markets in the general population (as do psychotherapeutic activities), the consultation practice field may be at a crucial juncture, both in regard to its survivability within the mental health professional community and in regard to its ability to capture a market segment capable of providing long-term fiscal sustenance through client fees. In the face of declining fiscal resources for the entire mental health field, in many agencies consultation may assume a low priority because of the perception that it cannot generate meaningful revenue for the "host" organization and that it may not appear to offer any new technological breakthrough that might be considered "revolutionary" or capable of rapidly capturing professional and public attention. In short, owing to forces substantially beyond its control, the field that originally nurtured the consultation movement may now be postured to either ignore or discredit its innovative offspring.

THE DEFINITION OF CONSULTATION

To *define* is to "determine or fix the boundaries or extent of" (*Random House*, 1967, p. 279). Establishing a definition of mental health consultation is important in that a fix on its boundaries will support and/or dictate other crucial factors. These include the extent and nature of the theory and ethics underlying practice; type, training, and auspice of consultants; and pragmatic considerations, such as clientele, funding, methodology, and the nature of variables to assess outcome.

Whether explicitly defined or illustrated through example and discussion, the many contexts and scope of mental health consultation as it is currently practiced have been described by the previous authors. The breadth and large range suggest the existence of myriad roles, anticipated outcomes, goals, and methods. These diverse expectations for consultation lead to questions of whether the boundaries of consultation have in fact been deliberately established to encompass a wide scope of activity or have not as yet been firmly fixed.

Taken collectively, the previous authors have portrayed consultation as an extension of clinical practice, a means for system change, a mental health prevention program, a mechanism for upgrading the quality of organization life, a strategy to provide indirect service to the community, and a mechanism for extending and coordinating existing services. If these visions are indeed capable of realization, the consultation field should now be in a position clearly to differentiate the assumptions, rationale, methods, applicability, and expected outcomes of either (1) a generic consultation model that would facilitate these outcomes or (2) several highly differentiated models of practice having limited, but nevertheless highly focused, applicability to a variety of unique circumstances.

Independent of the specific focus and purpose of any one consultation episode, the illustrations of consultation practice presented in this volume suggest that, in its most rudimentary form, consultation must be considered as one of the key helping processes in the mental health armamentarium. As such, the consultation process can be viewed as a relationship established between a person or persons who are dealing with an issue (the client or consultee) and others who are seeking to help resolve these issues via application of a conscious helping process. Thus identification of a particular ''style'' of consultation practice is predicated upon the content and context of the client's issues (e.g., a case episode with a patient, a difficult issue in the community) and upon the type of behavioral strategy the consultant utilizes.

As a whole, this volume's authors suggest at least four aspects of the consultation relationship that may apply to all forms of consultation. First, client-consultant relationships should be considered *voluntary:* both parties should have maximum degrees of freedom to explore issues without the impingement of external mandates. Second, the relationship is *temporary:* it is bounded by a set of timely issues that compose the focus of the consultation, and may be legitimately terminated at any stage in the process. Third, all forms of consultation should be *supportive* to the client. Finally, both parties must recognize the need for and build toward a *disciplined* relationship having clear and predictable working plans, standards, and criteria for monitoring the process as it unfolds. In this latter regard, the consultant has an ethical responsibility—and should have the skills—to articulate his or her model of consultation practice early in the entry phase of the process.

Whether the consultation episode be case, program, community-related, or some other type, the consultation model should illustrate the sequence of phases or other processes through which the consultant will guide the relationship and the attention to the client's issues. The consultant may advise that discussions of potential "solutions" to the client's situation can only follow a period of active listening in which both client and consultant attempt to accurately detail the parameters of the issue. Delineating a preferred activity sequence not only provides the client with a structure for addressing the issue; it also guides the consultant in consciously focusing interventions and behaviors. Thus both client and consultant simultaneously share the same knowledge regarding the purpose and context of the consultant's interventions at any particular point.

Such process "models" may take the form of guiding sequential questions, such as "What is wanted?" (determining client intents, goals, and objectives both for the consultation episode and for the client's entire problem situation), "What is?" (determining the current status quo and defining the situation more fully), and "What should be done?" (determining actions, actors, change strategies, the consultant's role, etc.) (see Pickering & Mazade, 1981). Other models might articulate specific sequential "phases" (e.g., entry, development of alternatives, problem solving, implementation, termination). Still others might describe specific episodes of the consultation process (Pattenaude & Landis, 1979); a series of client-consultant contracts (Milstein & Smith, 1979); overall guidelines for managing the process (Rehfuss, 1979); constructing new cognitive frameworks to define issues (Eiseman, 1978); engaging in a varied, creative, problem-solving process (DeBono, 1970); or articulating the specific steps in knowledge utilization (Sebring, 1979). Detailed models may even be developed for one specific element (e.g., entry) embedded within a larger model (Louis, 1980).

The need to define the scope of consultation and its various models clearly also becomes a crucial issue in evaluating the outcome of various consultation efforts. The paucity of well-formulated research designs undoubtedly stems from the inability of well-intentioned researchers/evaluators to understand the very phenomena being evaluated. The methodological difficulties in attempting to classify and understand the nature of consultation practice variables are illustrated in a study by Kaplan (1979) examining the relationships between consultation and improved client task performance. Efforts to construct evaluation taxonomies and their concomitant methodologies will be stymied until the field is able to provide clearly defined, describable, and observable paradigms of consultation practice (Perkins, 1977; Hoffman, 1979; Porrass & Berg, 1978; and Ganesh, 1978).

Intentionality

Of present consideration in the overall future both of consultation as a field of practice and/or of individual consultation episodes is intent. In considering the various definitions of consultation, its advent as a definable program entity in community mental health, and consultation's promise as a prevention strategy, the field might well examine the implications of these diverse expectations in relation to perceptions held by mental health consultants and (or versus) those of the client.

Given the extent to which the field has articulated desired intents and outcomes for mental health consultation, there may exist a potential danger both to preshape practice and to deliver an irrelevant service or product to clients. In their deliberate efforts to effect system change, to upgrade the level of community mental health, or to produce other outcomes described earlier, mental health consultation interventions may often be driven by larger, overarching goals to achieve outcomes not necessarily held or "owned" by the client. Thus various "models" and "types" may reflect the profession's valued goals (e.g., "prevention") instead of being explicitly designed to discover and deal with the client's agendas exclusively.

These issues would appear significant in relation to the consultant's perception of the client's "resistance," "health," "ability to admit problems," "hidden agendas," "displacement," and the like. If consultants initially hold salient goals, objectives, or expected outcomes different from those of the client, there would appear to exist a high potential for perceiving or labeling client behaviors in these terms. This situation is logical since the consultant is acting from one set of motivations, yet is in a situation of responding to client behaviors that originate from a completely different set of assumptions, norms, attitudes, thoughts, feelings, and expectations. Such a dilemma places individual mental health consultants (and the field as a whole) in a stance of either utilizing one's skills to achieve personally held values and outcomes (e.g., "increasing the quality of organizational life") or practicing "value-free" consultation in which consultants are committed to facilitating and helping to fulfill client-generated agendas that may or may not appear to have such altruistic intents.

The attitude toward and perception of "failure" is also closely related to these considerations. Numerous verbal and written accounts of unsuccessful consultation efforts often attribute such failure to the client's "inability to gain administrative support for the solution," impingement of "political realities," "language barriers" between consultant and client, or organizational policies that inhibit change and therefore maintain the problem situation. Yet it must be recognized that jargon, policy, administrative directives, and various constraints on the organization's relations with its environment (i.e., "politics") constitute essential constructs in maintaining the client's personal or organizational system. If consultants perceive these constructs to be the raison d'étre of failure in that they place unwarranted restrictions or controls on consultants, such a perception may suggest that consultants have not adequately included all components of the system in defining the issue and have not asked sufficient clarifying questions or otherwise attended to the client's intents for the consultation effort. In short, the discussions of failure often lament the fate of the *consultant's* recommendations, strategies, or problem-solving alternatives rather than those of the client.

SYSTEM ISSUES

Whether a consultant operates as an individual or from a multistaff organizational base, a variety of issues may arise within the consultant's system as well as in that of the client. Many of these intra- and intersystem issues have been illustrated by the previous authors and may be summarized here. Thompson (1975) suggested others.

To create and maintain a viable and supportive organizational base, the consultant's system should, at a minimum, develop and articulate the philosophy and rationale for undertaking consultation practice; have consensus from staff and governing board around the primary values inherent in this philosophy; formulate necessary administrative policies and procedures consistent with these values; have adequate training for consultants including opportunities for individual or group supervision; have developed adequate resources including sufficient funds, hours, skills, and energy; established a fee schedule; possess a record system that minimally reflects content, frequency, duration, goals, and stages in the consultation process; and have a process or procedure that will format data for purposes of evaluation, research, and accountability to both the consultant's organization and the client.

Likewise, clients have their own system needs to which they must attend independently or with the consultant's assistance. Clients should be in a position to clearly specify their need for consultation; they should also have an awareness of the available organizational resources for influencing the situation, have attempted to match issues to the type of consultant sought, and have a policy and administrative sanctions for participation in the consultation effort.

Issues at the interface between the two systems include those artifacts that evidence substantive work between the consultant and client or between members of their respective systems (e.g., business administrators of each system). The nature of these artifacts will, of course, depend on the nature of the consultation situation but might include a written statement of the client's perception of the issue; an "action plan" specifying goals, priorities, actors, and tasks to be accomplished; and/or a formal contract delineating several structural aspects of the consultation including purpose, time period, parties involved, description of the type of consultation, name of consultants and other providers, designation of the "clients," fees and method of payment, records, confidentiality provisions, grievance procedures, subcontracting provisions, and terms of modification (Mazade & Surles, 1976).

As demonstrated in this publication, one prerequisite for achieving a successful intervention is attention to the variety of system-level actors and the conditions that influence their behavior. This, in turn, may suggest the need for several multifaceted interventions to achieve change (Pasmore & King, 1978), many of which may be heavily dependent on the consultant's style (Lipshitz & Sherwood, 1978) and on the ability to achieve a psychologically symmetrical or egalitarian relationship with the client (Etzion, 1979) within an ethically acceptable framework (Pfeiffer & Jones, 1977).

SUMMARY

Most edited texts might conclude with a major section drawing attention to the major agreements (but more likely, the major conflicts) among the various contributors. Such is not the case here, for the wide potential scope of consultation practice has been described in a number of ways that do not inherently conflict, however, as the field moves toward a more detailed differentiation of process models in the next several years, conflicts among both practitioners and theoreticians may emerge. As the field begins to limit itself and become more sophisticated and experienced in providing focused services within limited settings, a reductionistic process is bound to occur in which highly specific theories, models, and outcome indicators will be proposed. Specific practice-based theories may be developed for "mental health consultation to schools" in which entry, data gathering, development of alternative interactions, and evaluation activities will be defined more as a "science" than as an "art." Concomitant issues regarding administration, consultant-client contracting, consultant training, institutionalizing of learnings, and other aspects of consultation in this particular setting may likewise be refined.

Forecasting the move toward greater specificity in mental health consultation reflects this author's hope and perception of this movement as an inevitable phenomenon. The authors in this volume appear to have identified the critical issues relevant to rapidly emerging technology. Through direct verbal or written observations of its leading practitioners, the scant research results that exist, feedback from former clients, and theoretical contributions from others in the behavioral sciences, the field has witnessed great strides in fulfillment of the three basic purposes of this book initially identified by the editors:

1. To understand the various dimensions of the behavioral role of the consultant and the process variables that influence it

2. To discuss aspects of improving consultation services to clients

3. To suggest indicators that can be utilized for monitoring consultation practice

Whether one focuses on models or on issues that influence day-to-day practice, or predicts the future of mental health consultation, these three goals must be satisfied in order to bring understanding and clarity to this burgeoning and most important field of mental health practice.

NOTE

1. The views expressed herein are solely those of the author and do not reflect the policy or views of the U.S. Department of Health and Human Services or the National Institute of Mental Health.

REFERENCES

Bowen, D. L., & Collett, M. J. When and how to use a consultant: Guidelines for public managers. *Public Administration Review,* 1978, *38,* pp. 476-481.

DeBono, E. *Lateral thinking: Creativity step by step.* New York: Harper Colophon Books, 1970.

Eiseman, J. W. Reconciling "incompatible" positions. *Journal of Applied Behavioral Science,* 1978, *14,* 133-150.

Etzion, D. Achieving balance in a consultation setting. *Group and Organization Studies,* 1979, *4,* 366-376.

Ganesh, S. R. Organizational consultants: A comparison of styles. *Human Relations,* 1978, *31,* 1-28.

Hoffman, L. R. Applying experimental research on group problem solving to organizations. *Journal of Applied Behavioral Science,* 1979, *15,375-391.*

Kaplan, R. E. The conspicuous absence of evidence that process consultation enhances task performance. *Journal of Applied Behavioral Science,* 1979, *15,* 346-360.

Lipshitz, R., & Sherwood, J. J. The effectiveness of third-party process consultation as a function of the consultant's prestige and style of intervention. *Journal of Applied Behavioral Science,* 1978, *14,* 493-509.

Louis, M. R. Surprise and sense making: What newcomers experience in entering unfamiliar organizational settings. *Administrative Science Quarterly,* 1980, *25,* 226-250.

Mazade, N., & Surles, R. *Considerations in the development of "fee for service" and "total cost" contracts for human service agencies* (mimeo). Chapel Hill, N.C.: Institute for Social Service Planning, 1976.

Milstein, M. M., & Smith, D. The shifting nature of OD contracts: A case study. *Journal of Applied Behavioral Science,* 1979, *15,* 179-191.

Pasmore, W. A., & King, D. C. Understanding organizational change: A comparative study of multifaceted interventions. *Journal of Applied Behavioral Science,* 1978, *14,* 455-468.

Pattenaude, R. L. Consultants in the public sector. *Public Administration Review,* 1979, 203-205.

————. & Landis, L. M. Consultants and technology transfer in the public sector. *Public Administration Review,* 1979, *39,* pp. 414-420.

Perkins, D. N. T. Evaluating social interventions: A conceptual schema. *Evaluation Quarterly,* 1977, *1,* 639-655.

Pfeiffer, J. W., & Jones, J. E. Ethical considerations in consulting. In *The 1977 annual handbook of group facilitators.* La Jolla, Calif.: University Associates, 1977, pp. 217-224.

Pickering, J., & Mazade, N. *Diagnostic questions and assumptions: Sequential contracts consultation model.* Unpublished workshop/training materials, 1981.

Porras, J. I., & Berg, P. O. Evaluation methodology in organization development: An analysis and critique. *Journal of Applied Behavioral Science,* 1978, *14,* 151-173.

————. *The Random House dictionary of the English language.* New York: Random House, 1967.

Rehfuss, J. Managing the consultantship process. *Public Administration Review,* 1979, *39,* pp. 211-214.

Sebring, R. H. Knowledge utilization in organization development. *Journal of Applied Behavioral Science,* 1979, *15,* 194-197.

Sterling, G. *Managing the public sector.* Homewood, Ill.: Dorsey Press, 1977.

Thompson, J. *Intersystem issues in the consultation relationship.* Unpublished training aid. Chapel Hill, N.C.: University of North Carolina School of Medicine, Division of Community Psychiatry, 1975.

INDEX

Individual process model
  and human service networks, 178,
    213–214, 219
  overview, 34–35, 57–69
Information systems
  community, 129–133
  program, 129, 130, 133–135
  requirements for, 128–129
Insurance reimbursements, 124
Integrity Groups, 194
Interpersonal skills (see Skills)
Intervention
  behavioral (see Educational-process
    model)
  criteria for, 140–141
  decision-making process, 141–150
  evaluating effectiveness of, 42, 45, 50
  implementation, 42, 49–50
  and program evaluation, 24
  strategies, 29–37, 44, 211, 212
    alternative designs, 85–87
  when not applicable, 68

Job Corps, 101
Joint Commission on Mental Illness and
  Health, 182, 183, 184

Law enforcement agencies
  behavior modification, 35
  as consultees, 20, 22, 67, 100–102,
    103, 123
    time available for consultation, 101
  and entry issues, 104, 108
  and gatekeeper role, 110
  and human service networks,
    178–179
  organizational procedures, 73, 75
  and termination, 115–116
Lay support networks (see Helping networks)
Levy, L.H., survey of mutual-help
  groups, 191
Lieber, Leonard, 193
Lindemann, Erich, 169
Linkages, concept of, 180, 206, 207
Low, Abraham, 193

McPheeters, Harold, 96
Maintenance subsystems, 74, 76, 78–80,
  83, 88
Management by objectives, 211–212
Management information system (see In-
  formation systems, program)
Management subsystems, 74, 76, 78–
  80, 83, 84, 88
Matrix model, 93

Mental health centers (see Community
  mental health centers)
Mental Health Demographic Profile Sys-
  tem (MHDPS), 131
Mental Health Study Center, 132
Mentally ill, reentry into society, 177,
  188–189, 190–191
Minority cultures, 177, 198–200
Modeling, 41, 43, 46, 48
Mutual-help groups, 176–177, 181, 185,
  186, 189–194, 198

Nader, Ralph, 127, 128
National health insurance program, 126
National Institute of Drug Abuse, 208
National Institute of Mental Health, 125,
  177, 191
National Self-Help Clearinghouse, 190,
  202
Natural helping networks (see Helping networks)
Neurotics Anonymous, 191
Norms, group
  changing, 85
  definition, 72–73
  formal, 74–75, 76, 80, 88
  informal, 76, 78, 80, 88
  and roles, 82–83, 84, 87, 88
  subsystems, 73–74
Nurses
  hospital, 20, 74, 77, 78, 123
  public health, 22, 67

Open-system model, 215–216

Parents Anonymous, 193
Parents Without Partners, 192
Peer reinforcement, 46–47
Peer supervision groups, 23
Personal feelings
  constructive use of, 58
  displacement technique, 59–61, 64
Phase models, 237
Police (see Law enforcement agencies)
Power (see also Management subsystems)
  creating, 97–98, 153, 156–162, 170
  distribution of, 175
  kinds, 153–154
  motives, 78, 88
  satisfactions, 79
  social, 158
President's Commission on Mental
  Health, 125, 126, 184–185, 190,
  191–192, 222
Prevention Council of the National Council of Community Health Centers, 96